NOURISH

mind, body & soul

Amber Rose grew up in New Zealand, surrounded by heritage fruit and vegetables in her mother's renowned organic permaculture garden. She is a food stylist and regularly cooks for clients in their homes (including Gwyneth Paltrow and Kate Hudson). In her cooking and baking, Amber focuses on produce-led, traditional diets and nutrient-dense foods and gets her inspiration from the seasons. Her first book was the best-selling *Love Bake Nourish*, which has been translated into five languages.

Sadie Frost lives in London with her four children. Apart from her roles for Fashion with Floozie and Iris and Edie by Frostfrench and her career as an actress, Sadie is currently involved with her film company Blonde to Black Pictures, which has just completed two feature films, with many more to come. Alongside this, Sadie has being working toward an MA with Raindance and Staffordshire University in Film Studies. She has always had a keen interest in health and fitness and has studied yoga, meditation, and nutrition for nearly 20 years. She recognizes that these things enable her to try to achieve the perfect balance to live calmly and to have a certain quality of peace of mind.

Holly Davidson grew up in the English countryside, beginning an active lifestyle from an early age. An established actor in film and television, she performed in dramatic and comedic roles for over ten years. Holly currently practices as a Level 3 personal trainer and fitness coach. Her numerous clients include celebrities Florence Welch, Nick Grimshaw, and Sienna Guillory. Renowned for her enthusiasm to motivate people, Holly is qualified in a range of techniques, such as kick-boxing, Pilates, kettle bells, TRX, and postnatal exercises, and consults on nutrition and lifestyle changes. She lives and works in London.

Amber
To my amazing and inspiring son and to all the beautiful, strong
women in my life, and to all the single parents out there—
you are all superheroes.

Sadie
To Fin, Raff, Iris, and Rudy, my little babies. And to my mother,
Mary Davidson, and grandmother, Betty Nolan, for being the most
nourishing women I've met.

Holly
To my wonderful mom and dad. Thank you for always believing in
me. I couldn't have chosen better.

NOURISH

Mind, body & soul

Amber Rose, Sadie Frost & Holly Davidson

Photography by David Loftus

Kyle Books

Published in 2015 by Kyle Books
www.kylebooks.com
general.enquiries@kylebooks.com

Distributed by National Book Network
4501 Forbes Blvd., Suite 200
Lanham, MD 20706
Phone: (800) 462-6420
Fax: (800) 338-4550

First published in Great Britain in 2014 by
Kyle Books, an imprint of Kyle Cathie Limited

ISBN 978-1-909487-32-1

Library of Congress Control Number: 2015939768

10 9 8 7 6 5 4 3 2 1

The information and advice contained in this book are
intended as a general guide. Neither the authors nor the
publishers can be held responsible for claims arising from
the inappropriate use of any remedy or exercise regime.
Do not attempt self-diagnosis or self-treatment for serious
or long-term conditions before consulting a medical
professional or qualified practitioner. Do not begin
any exercise program or undertake any self-treatment
while taking other prescribed drugs or receiving therapy
without first seeking professional guidance. Always seek
medical advice if any symptoms persist.

Text © Amber Rose, Sadie Frost & Holly Davidson 2014
Photographs © David Loftus 2014
Design © Kyle Books 2014

Author coordinator: Amber Rose
Copy editor: Stephanie Evans
Editorial assistant: Tara O'Sullivan
Proofreader: Catherine Ward
Americanizer: Christy Lusiak
Design: BuroCreative
Photographer: David Loftus

CONTENTS

INTRODUCTION

This is a book that covers health and nourishment for the mind, body, and soul.

We are three women, we are three friends, we are three people passionate about food, well-being, and exercise. In one way or another we have all been on a journey that has involved health issues and struggles with the pressures of life. In this book we share with you the tips, tricks, solutions, and answers that we have learned along the way to get our bodies back in shape, to get our health back on track after illness, to still our minds among the stresses of family and life, or just to maintain a positive and happy outlook and, above all, to have fun.

For each of us, this book is about sharing information among women, families, and generations. It's about wisdom and nourishment. It's about community and coming together to support each other to lead the happiest and best lives we can, to feel that we have a few tricks up our sleeves and tools in our tool box—so that even when obstacles block our path, we have the knowledge and support to get over them, around them, or under them and back on track.

The book is arranged into three major sections: food, mind, and body, with Holly Davidson bringing you amazing exercise routines and plans to strengthen and inspire, to get you motivated, or to push you through to the next level to up your game. Holly's enthusiasm is infectious and inspiring and her exercise programs are easy to follow with fantastic results.

In Sadie Frost's section, you will find her sharing her gorgeous home beauty recipes and remedies to soothe tired skin, to bring a shine back to your hair, or simply to pamper yourself after a grueling week. Sadie also shares her knowledge of meditation, yoga, and mindfulness to encourage peace of mind and contentment. Such useful tools for anyone to have.

Amber Rose shares the recipes that she uses on a daily basis to support health and happiness. They are seasonal, nutrient-dense recipes that can be cooked to nourish the body, strengthen the immune system, and heal a stressed digestive system. They are the recipes that she cooks for family and friends during a busy week, a lazy weekend breakfast, or a big celebration; whatever the occasion, there is always a way to stay healthy and keep it delicious.

In this book, we hope that you find knowledge, support, and nourishment that will help you on your journey, as it has ours. Enjoy.

Love,
Amber, Sadie & Holly x

SUPERFOOD

Amber

I enjoyed a free-range childhood, spending my days eating and cooking from my mother's garden, picking wild flowers, and foraging for wild fruits and berries and other delights. I would happily forsake a clean dress if it meant I could just reach that ripest, juiciest, and most delicious blackberry at the very top of the prickliest and highest cane. I have always loved eating, but have also loved the process of gathering, collecting, and preparing the food. The ingredients we gather and cook are what sustain us and those we love.

Food is such an integral part of lives, families, and greater communities. It can define who we are, how we relate to one another, and how we feel about ourselves. I love the way food can bring people together. Community has always been a big thing for me. I am connected to those around me, the people I love, through expression, and one of the ways I express myself is through food. Food can be warming, earthy, and robust—exactly what we need for those cold winter months when days are short and we need comfort and sustenance of the highest order—or it can be light, delicate, gentle, restorative, or cleansing for the warmer lighter spring and summer months. The way we eat greatly determines how we feel about ourselves. It's easy to forget that sometimes. Food is medicine

Food is such an integral part of lives, families, and greater communities. It can define who we are, how we relate to one another, and how we feel about ourselves.

and medicine is food. The idea that we can adapt what and how we eat to alter how we feel within ourselves is empowering. My style of cooking and baking is produce led and based on traditional diets with nutrient-dense foods, healthy fats, and heritage produce. This is how my mother cooked for me, and how I choose to cook for my family and those I love. Making nourishing meals is serious business, but that doesn't mean it can't also be playful, easy to prepare, and above all, a pleasure to eat and share with those around you.

I have never had any formal training. I am a self-taught cook, but I have had a passion and a love for good food passed down to me by a mother who has one of the most wonderful gardens in New Zealand, filled with over 800 varieties of fruits and vegetables, and a father who was a chef. Our pantry was my mother's garden, a giant, open-air cupboard, if you like. As a little girl, I would find things in my mother's vegetable patch to harvest and cook. Over the years, that hasn't really changed much—there's a very seasonal and flexible approach to creating my menus; my style of cooking is very simple, with lots of fresh herbs thrown in for good measure. And what I feed my son is what I eat myself. He is a great eater and I feel that is partly because I choose to eat with him and we always share

that moment of the day together. From an early age, he would pick bits of salad off my plate and try new things because he saw me enjoying it so he thought he would give it a try. Mealtimes should be shared and always a pleasure. This is how children grow to love and understand food.

The inspiration for me to write this book has been based on my feelings about families, community, friends, sharing, loving, learning, and growing. I find it quite wonderful that three friends can come together to share what they have learned from different walks of life to support one another, as well as women everywhere so that we can all support ourselves and our families.

I am a single parent and without my community of friends around me, I wouldn't be where I am today. For me, this book is about sharing with you what I have learned along the way—from that free-range childhood through to supporting women through childbirth as a doula, and from being a mom myself to being a friend and someone who loves to share my knowledge and support with anyone who wants it.

Lots of love,
Amber x

SMOOTHIES

&

JUICES

This chapter includes juices, smoothies, delicious fruity waters, hot drinks, and my favorite hot chocolate of all time—you just won't believe it tastes so good and is also so good for you!

Juices and smoothies are a great way to start the morning. A big breakfast doesn't usually work for me during the week when I'm busy and rushing around, so I often have a juice or a smoothie for breakfast instead. Juices and smoothies are really cleansing and nourishing. They are a great way of getting all the nutrients and energy that you need for your morning without the heavy feeling a big breakfast can give you if you're busy and up early. Don't get me wrong though, I love big breakfasts! I just usually save them for the weekend and turn them into a leisurely affair.

I spent my childhood wandering through my mother's gardens, picking herbs and flowers for tea and always choose a fresh herbal tea over a dried one. Fresh herbal tea is so easy to make, and if you have herbs in your garden or even some dried herbs in jars, you can make up combos that suit what you feel like. I love adding lemon or lime to pots of fresh herbal tea. Fresh tea has a lot more going for it than anything you will get from a bag, and it's just as quick and easy. Of course, there are moments when nothing but a perfectly brewed cup of Earl Grey tea will do, and on those occasions I love

nothing more than a pot with some raw milk or my favorite homemade almond milk, sweetened with a touch of honey— tastes like perfection!

The two biggest benefits to making your own juices and smoothies are that 1) they taste amazing, much better than anything you can buy in a bottle; and 2) because they are freshly made from whole fruit and not packaged, they have not been pasteurized, as pretty much all juices and smoothies you will find on a supermarket shelf have been. The process of pasteurization kills off all the beneficial enzymes, which are what helps you digest any of the goodness in the fruit or vegetables. When you buy bottled juices and smoothies, you are pretty much just drinking sugar, unless they are cold pressed, unpasteurized, and very fresh.

Another good thing to remember is that by adding kefir or full-fat coconut milk to smoothies, you are adding the "good fats" that make all the micronutrients bioavailable. To get around this when juicing, I always add some good seed or nut oils to my fresh juices, or even some cod liver oil—there are some great brands out there that don't have a fishy taste but do provide you with your essential fatty acids. So there you have it, a few great reasons why making your own drinks is not only super delicious but also nourishing and rewarding for your body.

A DELICIOUS GREEN SMOOTHIE

This is my favorite smoothie; it's simply the goodness of the greens. Perfection.

1 small banana, sliced and frozen ahead of time
Handful of spinach or kale
1 scoop of your favorite powdered super greens
1 teaspoon raw coconut oil
1 teaspoon fish oils or your favorite omega oil
1 teaspoon raw honey
1¼ cups filtered water, almond milk, or coconut water

Place all the ingredients in a blender and process until completely smooth.

SUPER RED BERRY & KEFIR SMOOTHIE

Milk kefir is so full of probiotics and enzymes and it has a wonderful slightly sour, tangy taste, which balances with the berries perfectly. Kefir helps with digestion and supports the immune system. This is a great smoothie for both kids and adults.

1 cup milk kefir
1 tablespoon raw honey
1 teaspoon raw coconut oil
½ large banana, previously frozen, sliced
Handful of any frozen red berries (strawberries or raspberries work well)
1 heaping tablespoon goji berries, soaked overnight in filtered water and drained

Put everything into a blender and process for 2 minutes or until completely smooth.

Drink and enjoy.

BLACKBERRY, ROSE & RAW CHOCOLATE SMOOTHIE

This smoothie is great for kids and adults. You may want to leave out the rose water for the kids, though; it's quite a grown-up flavor, but a delightful one for those who love it!

1 large banana
Large handful of frozen blackberries
1 heaping teaspoon raw coconut oil
1 teaspoon raw honey
1 teaspoon rose water
2 teaspoons raw cacao powder
1 cup almond milk
½ teaspoon cacao nibs (optional), to serve

Place all of your prepared ingredients into a blender and process for 2 minutes or until completely smooth.

Pour into a glass and sprinkle with the cacao nibs, (if using).

Red berries are full of antioxidants.

BANANA & ALMOND SMOOTHIE

with Cinnamon

This is a wonderful smoothie. I usually have a few frozen bananas kicking around in my freezer and cinnamon is a staple in the pantry, so it's easy to rustle up and is one that both adults and kids love. Cinnamon is great for curbing sweet cravings and pairs beautifully with the banana.

1 large banana, previously frozen, sliced
1¼ cups almond milk
1 hearty teaspoon almond butter
1 teaspoon raw coconut oil
¼ teaspoon cinnamon
½ teaspoon raw honey

Toppings to serve
Handful of soaked raw almonds,
  drained and coarsely chopped (optional)
A dusting of cinnamon

Process all the ingredients in a blender until smooth. Pour into a glass and sprinkle with a little extra cinnamon and some chopped nuts, if you like.

MEAN GREEN MORNING SMOOTHIE

with Extra Protein

Protein is an important part of your diet and nuts are a really good source, especially for vegetarians and vegans.

1 small handful of soaked raw almonds or cashews
1 tablespoon almond butter
2 medjool dates, pitted
4 kale leaves, stalks removed and chopped
1 teaspoon of your favorite powdered super greens
1 cup kefir or unsweetened almond milk
1 large handful of ice cubes

Simply place everything into a blender and process for 2 minutes, or until completely smooth. For a thinner consistency, add a little more kefir, almond milk, or water and blend again.

BEET KVASS

Beet Kvass, an inexpensive health tonic that is made from fermented beets, has powerful medicinal qualities and acts as a digestive aid. Beets are packed full of nutrients. One small glass in the morning and night is an excellent blood tonic; it promotes regularity, aids digestion, alkalizes the blood, cleanses the liver, and is a good treatment for kidney stones and other ailments. It has a wonderful savory, earthy, slightly sour, and tangy flavor. Before I tried this I wasn't expecting to like it, but I love beets and it quickly grew on me. Now I love it, and would even go so far as to say I crave it!

Makes about a half gallon

2–4 beets, depending on size, washed, peeled, and diced into ¾ in cubes

3 tablespoons whey★ (see right)

1 tablespoon sea salt or Himalayan salt (not table salt)

Filtered water (not tap water: the chlorine will prevent fermentation)

A large half gallon jar or jug, sterilized (boil for 10 minutes on the rack of a boiling-water canner)

Place the diced beets in the bottom of your glass jar. Add the whey and salt, then fill the jar with filtered water. Cover with a kitchen towel or cheesecloth and leave on the counter for two days to ferment. Transfer the whole jar, with a tight-fitting lid, to the fridge.

To drink, simply ladle off a small amount—roughly ⅓ cup—morning and night. When the liquid is finished, you can eat the beets at the bottom if you like; these are now what you call lacto-fermented vegetables. The Beet Kvass will last well for several months in the fridge, by which time you will most likely have polished it off.

★ To make whey, simply place about 1½ cups of plain unsweetened yogurt (not Greek yogurt) in a cheesecloth, tie it up, and hang it over a bowl. I do this in my sink and tie the cheesecloth to the tap with a piece of string. The thin white liquid that starts to drip from the bottom is whey. By adding whey to the Beet Kvass mix you will stop any unfriendly bacteria from growing. The leftover plain yogurt is now like Greek yogurt, which is delicious.

It has powerful medicinal qualities and acts as a digestive aid.

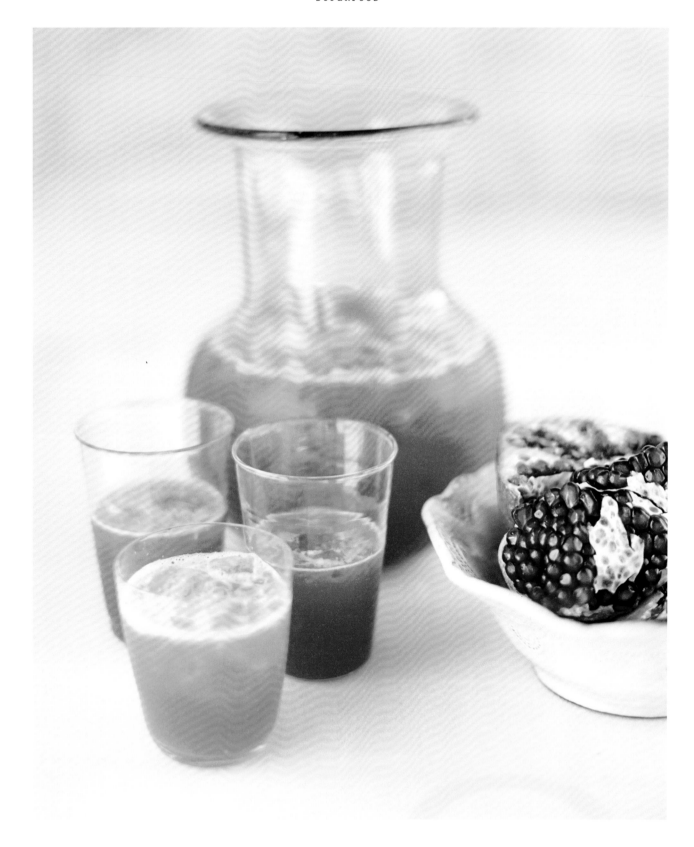

BLOOD ORANGE, POMEGRANATE & GRAPEFRUIT JUICE

This beautifully colored drink is packed full of anthocyanins, which are powerful antioxidants that come from the intense color of the blood oranges and the pinks in the grapefruits and the dark reds of the pomegranate. It's a special treat when blood oranges are in season.

4 blood oranges, peeled and quartered
Seeds from 1 pomegranate
½ pink grapefruit, peeled and halved
¼ lemon, peeled

Wash and prepare your fruit, put through the juicer, and drink immediately.

GREEN JUICE

This green juice is nourishing, cleansing, and delicious. The mint really lifts the flavor and gives it a refreshing zing.

1 green apple
½ cucumber
½ fennel bulb
Handful of kale
1 kiwi fruit, peeled
3 sprigs of mint
3 stems of parsley
¼ lemon, peeled
Small piece of fresh ginger, peeled

Wash all the ingredients, put everything through a juicer, and drink immediately.

ABC

with Ginger & Turmeric

I love having a juice before 10am when the liver is in full cleanse mode. Juicing first thing helps your system to cleanse, refresh, and start fully loaded with enzymes and immune-supporting goodness. If you can't find fresh turmeric, use a pinch of turmeric powder.

1 apple
1 medium beet
6 carrots
Small piece of fresh ginger, peeled
Small piece of fresh turmeric, peeled
¼ lemon, peeled
1 teaspoon of your favorite omega or fish oils
Freshly cracked black pepper

Wash all the fruit and vegetables and put through the juicer. Add the oils and a twist of black pepper. Drink immediately.

GINGER TEA

with Honey

This is the simplest of teas, but so good and so easy. It's alkalizing and perfect throughout the day.

A few slices of fresh ginger, peeled
1 teaspoon raw honey

Bring a pot of water to a boil, fill your tea cup or mug, and gently place the slices of ginger into the steaming water. Let sit for a minute or two before adding the honey.

ALKALIZING CIDER VINEGAR TEA

with Raw Honey

This is a great tea to start the day with. It's very alkalizing and is good for flushing the liver.

1 teaspoon unpasteurized raw apple cider vinegar
1 teaspoon raw honey

Simply bring a pot of water to a boil, fill your tea cup, and let it sit for a minute or two to cool before stirring in the vinegar and honey. (By allowing the water to cool a little, you will avoid destroying the health properties of the vinegar and honey.) Stir and drink.

MINT & ORANGE BLOSSOM TEA

Both mint and orange are uplifting, so this will elevate your mood and bring general cheer. It's also cleansing and delicious.

6 fresh or dried mint leaves
6 fresh or dried orange blossoms
Raw honey to taste (optional)

Place the herb leaves and flowers into a large teapot and pour in boiling water.

Allow to steep for 6–7 minutes. You can add honey if you like, to taste. I prefer it without, but that's just me…

Very delicious

HOT CHOCOLATE

This delicious hot chocolate has all the allure and taste of hot chocolate but without any of the nastiness contained in the more conventional sugar-laden type. It has cacao, which is FULL of mood-enhancing properties and wonderful antioxidants. It's full of healthy fats, which feed the brain and give energy without being stored. It has natural sweetening, and above all, it is still comforting and delicious. Such a treat for a rainy cold day, when a blanket and a cozy spot with a mug of this is the only thing that will give warmth and deliciousness.

Small handful of cashew nuts, soaked in filtered water for a few hours or overnight
1¾ cups full-fat coconut milk
1½ tablespoons raw cacao powder
1 tablespoon raw honey or raw date syrup (see page 119), (or to taste—you can add more after it is heated if you want it sweeter)

Optional flavorings:
Pinch of cinnamon
¼ teaspoon orange zest
or
¼ teaspoon vanilla powder
or
Pinch of chile powder and a pinch of cinnamon

Drain and rinse the soaked cashews.

Throw everything into a blender, including the extra spices, if you like. Process until you have a smooth liquid.

Pour it into a saucepan and place over gentle heat until it reaches your desired temperature. Taste for sweetness and add more honey or date syrup, if you wish.

CUCUMBER, MINT, LIME & KIWI WATER

This is a cleansing, refreshing way to get your fluids in the hot summer months. You can prepare this the night before so it's ready the next morning. To make it extra cold, just add a handful of ice.

½ **cucumber, sliced**
6 **sprigs mint**
3 **limes, sliced**
2 **kiwi fruit, peeled and sliced**
2 **quarts pure spring or mineral water**
   or freshly filtered water

Put all the ingredients into a large jug and let sit in a cool place or the fridge for at least 30 minutes.

RED SUMMER BERRIES
with Lemon & Rose

This is such a beautiful way to drink water, infused with the scent of rose and strawberries and the taste of lemon. It has extra cleansing properties from the lemon and berries. It's best drunk within one day, but, if I'm really thirsty or sharing this with others, I drink all the water and then keep topping it off throughout the day. You can add ice to keep it cool.

2½ **cups mixed red berries**
   (strawberries and raspberries work well)
2 **lemons, sliced**
2 **big garden roses, washed and petals removed**
   (must be unsprayed)
2 **quarts pure spring or mineral water**
   or freshly filtered water

Put all the ingredients into a large jug and let sit in a cool place or the fridge for at least 30 minutes. You could also make this the night before so it's ready to go the next morning.

TO START THE DAY

breakfast

Breakfasts are often the highlight of my day. I am a HUGE breakfast fan, and love everything from making my own granolas to pancakes and healthy homestyle breakfasts (if you can believe it's possible, which it is!!!). My son LOVES breakfasts too. During the week, I try to be organized and have some kind of seasonal fruit compôte in the fridge that I can add to oatmeal or to yogurt and granola. Whether it's a quick weekday start or a leisurely weekend affair, there is every reason to prepare something beautiful, seasonal, delicious, and nutrient-dense. In this chapter, I hope you will find lots of inspiration and new ideas to try out.

LEMON & POPPY SEED SWEET OMELET

Here's a refreshing way to start any day! The tart lemon lifts and adds a brightness, the poppy seeds provide a tasty little crunch, and what could be better than maple syrup and berries? The omelet is grain-free and full of essential good fats to feed your brain for a busy day ahead. It can easily be dairy-free if you use coconut yogurt, which is so good for you and utterly delicious.

Serves 1
2 free-range eggs
Pinch of good salt
1 generous teaspoon maple syrup,
   plus extra for drizzling
Zest of ¼ lemon,
   plus extra to serve
1 teaspoon poppy seeds
1 heaping teaspoon coconut oil

To serve
1 generous dollop of your favorite yogurt
1 small handful of fresh blueberries

Place a small frying pan over medium–high heat. Break the eggs into a small bowl and whisk thoroughly until they are very light and fluffy: the fluffier the eggs, the fluffier your omelet. Mix in the salt, syrup, lemon zest, and half the poppy seeds.

Add the coconut oil to the hot pan, letting it cover the bottom, then use a flat wooden spatula to spread it around. When the oil is hot, pour in your egg mixture. Let cook for a minute or two before carefully pulling in the sides with the spatula while tilting the pan, letting the egg run back out to fill the gap. Continue in this fashion until there is no runny mix left. Now carefully flip the omelet over—the second side will only need 30 seconds or so.

Gently slide the omelet out of the pan onto a waiting plate, spoon over your favorite yogurt, and top with blueberries and a final drizzle of maple syrup. Sprinkle with the remaining poppy seeds and some lemon zest. Enjoy while hot.

COCONUT &
BANANA PANCAKES

I love pancakes (who doesn't?)! These little ones are great topped with fresh fruit and yogurt for breakfast or brunch, or served as an afternoon snack. Sounds naughty but it doesn't have to be if you use organic cream or whipped coconut cream sweetened with honey and a fresh sugar-free berry jam—then everything is good for you and totally nourishing.

Serves 2–3

2 ripe medium bananas, coarsely chopped
4 whole eggs
2 tablespoons honey
¾ cup unsweetened, dried coconut flakes
1 cup almond meal
½ teaspoon gluten-free baking powder
Coconut oil or ghee

To serve

A few spoonfuls of your favorite yogurt
Handful of your favorite seasonal fruit
Toasted coconut or cacao nibs

Put the bananas, eggs, and honey in a food processor and purée until light and fluffy (or use a bowl and an immersion blender). Add the coconut, almond meal, and baking powder and beat to combine.

Heat up a tiny amount of coconut oil or ghee in your frying pan over low–medium heat. Cook in batches, allowing a large spoonful of mix per pancake—too big and they are really hard to flip, so keep them on the small size. Cook thoroughly—they should take about 1½ minutes on each side; you will know when to flip them once little bubbles start to appear on the surface. Keep warm and continue to cook the rest of the batter, adding a little more oil to the pan between batches.

Serve while hot and delicious, with some of your favorite toppings.

POACHED EGGS

with Cauliflower Toasts,
Kale & Dukkah

This delicious ensemble is a serious treat—one of my all-time favorites. Cauliflower toasts
give the poached eggs something to sit on and add texture without the need for bread.

Serves 2
1 whole cauliflower, outer leaves removed
3 tablespoons cold-pressed olive oil
5 tablespoons Dukkah (see page 115) or lightly
   crushed cumin seeds, plus extra to serve
2 tablespoons cold-pressed olive oil
1 tablespoon butter
2 garlic cloves, thinly sliced
½ medium red chile (optional), finely sliced
6–8 kale or cavolo nero leaves, on the large side,
   center stalks stripped out
4 free-range eggs
Pinch of salt

To serve
Cold-pressed extra virgin olive oil
Juice of ½ lemon
A few twists of black pepper

Preheat the oven to 400°F and line a baking sheet with parchment paper. Cut the cauliflower across into four slices of "toast" about ½–¾ in thick. Drizzle with 3 tablespoons of the oil, sprinkle with dukkah, place the toasts on your pan, and pop into the oven for about 30 minutes until they start to turn lovely and golden.

After 20 minutes, melt the remaining 2 tablespoons oil and butter in a medium casserole or Dutch oven with a lid over medium heat. Add the garlic and chile (if using), stir for 30 seconds, add the kale, then a few tablespoons of water, and a pinch of salt. Cover tightly with the lid and braise for 10 minutes, stirring occasionally. You may need to turn the heat down or add a little extra water if it is cooking too furiously.

Place a wide, deep saucepan over high heat and fill it with boiling water. Bring it to a light simmer and add a pinch of salt. Carefully crack one egg into a cup then gently pour it into the simmering water. Repeat with the remaining eggs and cook to your liking. Depending on their size, a soft-poached egg takes about 2 minutes and a soft to firm one needs about 4 minutes.

When everything is ready, place the cauliflower toasts onto warm plates, top with the eggs, and place the kale alongside. Sprinkle with a little extra dukkah and drizzle with cold-pressed extra virgin olive oil, then squeeze some lemon over the kale and season with a few twists of pepper.

ONE PLAIN OMELET

You can add any number of things to make it into something filling and satisfying. One of my favorite ways to serve an omelet is with plenty of sorrel, which can sometimes be found in organic grocery stores or farmers' markets. It is full of calcium and magnesium—two things we could all do with more of. I love the sourness of sorrel. Omelets go well with roast sweet potato or squash and a green salad. Steamed greens work well with plenty of good grass-fed butter and some quality sea salt.

Serves 1
Small pat of butter or odorless coconut oil
2 eggs, lightly beaten
Sea salt flakes and freshly cracked black pepper

A few good things to have with an omelet:
• **A few slices of avocado**
• **A sprinkle of your favorite herb**
• **Cheese, grated onto the omelet just before
  you fold it in half**
• **Radish Salad with Lemon & Parsley (see page 53)**
• **A few cherry tomatoes, pan-fried
  with butter and thyme**
• **Any kind of steamed green: kale, broccoli, etc.**
• **A few green leaves—kale or Romaine, lightly
  dressed with lemon juice and olive oil**
• **Baby spinach, wilted in a hot pan with a tiny
  bit of butter or oil**
• **A sprinkle of Dukkah (see page 115)**

Add your pat of butter or coconut oil to the pan and as soon as it sizzles, pour in the egg. After a minute or two, carefully tilt the pan and use a flat wooden spatula to pull in the sides of the omelet and then let it go—the egg will run back out to the sides filling the gap. Do this a few times around the pan, then let it cook for a few moments. When nearly all the egg is set, gently flip and fold over one side, slide it onto a waiting plate, and eat immediately.

OATMEAL

*with Fresh Summer Berries, Lemon Zest,
Maple Syrup & Toasted Coconut*

*Although oatmeal is generally thought of as a warming breakfast for winter,
I sometimes enjoy it as a summer dish too, served with fresh fruit, which
makes it lighter, and summer berries add a zingy, fresh taste. This is totally
scrumptious and very nourishing.*

Serves 2
1¼ cups whole rolled oats
**2 cups unsweetened almond milk
  or spring water**
¼ teaspoon finely grated lemon zest
Pinch of salt

To serve
½ cup shredded coconut
Yogurt of choice
**2 big handfuls of summer berries
  of your choice (I like to use
  blueberries and raspberries)**
Maple syrup to taste

First toast your coconut. Place a large frying pan over medium heat and let it warm up for a few minutes until you can feel the heat coming off the pan. Pour in the coconut and stir constantly with a wooden spoon. Slowly, it will start to turn a lovely golden brown but if it doesn't start to color, you need to turn up the heat. Once it's golden and smells delicious, transfer it into a waiting bowl to cool.

To make your oatmeal, put the oats, milk or water, lemon zest, and salt into a saucepan and place over medium–high heat. Bring to a boil. Once it bubbles, stir constantly with a wooden spoon for 5–6 minutes. Remove the pan from the heat and divide between 2 bowls.

Serve with a generous dollop of your favorite yogurt, then scatter with the fresh berries, drizzle with the maple syrup, and top with the toasted coconut. Enjoy.

BUCKWHEAT OATMEAL

with Cinnamon & Golden raisins

This is just the thing to keep you nourished and balanced. It's a bowl of such delicious flavors that you'll be in breakfast heaven—I sometimes even have this for dessert. Blackberries and pears are the perfect fruit combination for fall and winter since they're full of antioxidants, gentle on the digestive system, and yet full of fiber, vitamins C and E, and other essential nutrients. Cinnamon is a warming spice, great for curbing sugar cravings, and the thyme adds a delicious sweet note. Despite its name, buckwheat is technically not a grain but a seed. It is gluten-free with a lovely nutty flavor and it has a natural affinity with pears.

Serves 2

1¼ cup buckwheat groats
¼ teaspoon cinnamon
Small handful of golden raisins
Small handful of blackberries
1 cup spring water
2 cups unsweetened almond milk,
   or your favorite raw milk
Pinch of good salt

To serve
2 big dollops of yogurt of your choice
1 ripe pear, peeled, cored, and sliced
   lengthwise into quarters
Maple syrup to taste
Small handful of roasted and roughly
   chopped almonds
A few sprigs of thyme (optional but delicious)

Put the buckwheat, cinnamon, raisins, and blackberries in a saucepan with the water, bring to a boil, and then reduce the heat to a very gentle simmer. As the buckwheat start to absorb the water, stir in half the almond milk. Cover with a lid and allow the groats to absorb more of the liquid. You will need to stir the pan regularly with a wooden spoon and, when the buckwheat has absorbed almost all the milk, add the rest of the milk and a pinch of salt, stir thoroughly, replace the lid, and allow them to absorb the rest of the liquid. The whole process should take 20–30 minutes—you may need to add a little more liquid if the buckwheat starts to dry out before they have finished cooking, so keep an eye on the pan.

When it is ready, divide the oatmeal between two bowls, top with yogurt and the pear quarters, then drizzle with maple syrup and sprinkle with the chopped almonds and some thyme, if you wish.

GRANOLA

Grain-free with Rose water,
Apricot & Pistachio

This is a heavenly, fruity, floral combination. It's quite a decadent granola and not cheap to make; however, it lasts a long time and is not the kind of granola you would have a huge bowl of. I tend to serve it sprinkled on top of fresh fruit and yogurt. It looks so pretty and adds crunch and flavor to what you serve it with. It's full of slow-release energy and is super easy to make.

Makes 1 large jar
¼ **cup raw coconut oil**
⅓ **cup honey**
⅓ **cup maple syrup**
2 **cups coconut chips**
1 **cup pistachios, coarsely chopped**
1 **cup almonds, very coarsely chopped**
¾ **cup sunflower seeds**
½ **cup pumpkin seeds**
1 **teaspoon rose water (optional)**
1½ **cups dried apricots, coarsely chopped**
2 **tablespoons hemp seeds**
2–3 **tablespoons dried rose petals (optional)**

Preheat the oven to 325°F and line two deep-sided baking sheets with parchment paper. Melt the coconut oil, honey, and maple syrup in a small saucepan until it starts to bubble and simmer, then turn off the heat.

Combine the coconut chips, pistachios, almonds, and sunflower and pumpkin seeds in a large bowl. Pour in the honey mixture and stir with a wooden spoon until thoroughly combined. There should be enough of the honey mixture to lightly coat all the dry mix, but if you feel there is not enough, just add more honey mix using equal amounts of melted honey and coconut oil.

Spread the mixture onto the lined baking sheets, making a layer that isn't too deep, otherwise it won't all crisp up. Bake for 15–20 minutes, stirring every 3–4 minutes so that all the mix turns a lovely golden color and doesn't burn, which it can do easily due to the coconut. Remove from the oven, let cool a little, then sprinkle with the rose water (if using) and scatter in the dried apricots and hemp seeds. Lastly, stir through the petals (if using).

Let cool completely before transferring into an airtight jar. Use within two weeks.

MY NOURISHING OVERNIGHT BERRY & CHIA PARFAIT

This is a delicious breakfast that will give you a jump start to the day. I don't always like to eat first thing in the morning, so when I have to be up early for work, this is an ideal way to have a healthy breakfast on the go. Sometimes I make this the night before and put it in the fridge in a small jar with a tight-fitting lid, allowing enough room at the top to add yogurt and fruit once the parfait has set. For the more leisurely breakfast, layer it in a beautiful glass, starting with a layer of the parfait, followed by a layer of yogurt, then a layer of fruit, then a sprinkling of Granola (see page 40). The kids like to get involved in this too.

Serves 2
For the parfait:
1½ cups of your favorite milk
**¾ cup dark berries (use a mix of
    raspberries, strawberries, and blueberries)**
6 tablespoons chia seeds
1 tablespoon raw coconut oil
Drizzle of maple syrup or raw honey

To serve (any or all of the following)
Small handful of fresh berries
Your favorite yogurt
Seeds from ½ pomegranate
2 tablespoons shelled hemp seeds
Cacao nibs
Chopped nuts

Put all the ingredients for the parfait into a blender and process until thoroughly combined. Spoon one third of the mixture into the bottom of a glass and another third into the bottom of a second glass and the remaining third into a spare small container. Put all three in the fridge to set overnight.

When you are ready to eat this glass of delicious goodness, take both glasses from the fridge, sprinkle over some berries, then layer some yogurt and half of the remaining chia parfait into each glass. Top with more fresh fruit and any of the suggested toppings.

AVOCADO, BASIL & RED
PEPPER FLAKES ON TOAST

*This has to be one of my easiest and yet most delicious recipes. It's certainly one that
I make most frequently—for breakfast, brunch (with a poached egg), lunch (with
two eggs), and sometimes for dinner when I'm too busy to cook… It's AMAZING
sprinkled with a little dukkah, and also so good for you—full of healthy fats and essential
micronutrients that support your immune system and general health.*

Serves 2
1 avocado
¼ teaspoon red pepper flakes
6 basil leaves, torn
3 tablespoons really good extra virgin olive oil
Squeeze of lemon juice
Sea salt and freshly ground black pepper

For the toast:
**A couple of slices of your favorite toast—perhaps
    sourdough rye or Cauliflower Toasts (see page 34)**
1 garlic clove, halved
2 tablespoons good olive oil

To serve
Dukkah (see page 115), (optional)

Slice the avocado in half and remove the pit. Use a small
sharp knife to slice the inside of the avocado into large
squares without cutting into the skin. Now take a spoon
and scoop out the squares and put them in a bowl,
along with the red pepper flakes, torn basil leaves, and
oil. Squeeze over the lemon, add some salt and pepper
to taste, and give it a good but gentle stir—you don't
want mush.

Toast the bread and rub it all over with half a garlic
clove—I like it really garlicky, but if you prefer it less so,
just give a very light rub with the garlic. Drizzle with
some good oil and sprinkle with a little sea salt and a
few twists of pepper. Top with the avocado and serve
with dukkah (if using).

MY SPICE-SCENTED
HOMEMADE BEANS ON TOAST

*I love beans on toast, and this is a version that I've been making for years.
Kids love it too. Either serve them simply as beans on a nice piece of toasted
sourdough rye or on Cauliflower Toasts (see page 34) if you want to go grain-free.
This is delicious served alongside lightly-steamed kale, a delicious soft-poached egg,
or roasted veggies.*

Serves 4–6

3 tablespoons cold-pressed olive oil
2 medium onions, coarsely chopped
2 garlic cloves, grated or finely chopped
½ teaspoon ground cumin
½ teaspoon whole cumin seeds
1 × 14 oz can chopped tomatoes
1 tablespoon tomato paste
½ cup maple syrup
⅓ cup apple cider vinegar
1 cup water
2 × 14 oz cans white beans
   (cannellini or navy beans), rinsed and drained
Salt and pepper to taste

To serve
A few slices of your favorite cheese
A few sprigs of cilantro
½ medium red chile, seeded and finely sliced

Heat the oil in a large, heavy-bottomed casserole
or saucepan, add the onion, garlic, and cumin, and
stir for 3–5 minutes, or until the onion is translucent
and softened.

Add the canned tomatoes, the tomato paste, maple
syrup, vinegar, and water. Bring to a boil, add the beans,
reduce the heat to very low, and let simmer gently,
uncovered, for about 1½ hours: you will need
to stir the beans regularly and add more water if they
are drying out. After this time the beans should be
lovely and soft and the sauce should be wonderfully
thick. Season to taste.

Sometimes, if I am feeling really decadent, I add a few
shavings of my favorite cheese or sprinkle some cilantro
and chile on top. Whatever you decide, enjoy this while
it's hot.

SOM TUM POLLAMAI

Seasonal Fruit Salad with
Thai Herbs & Fresh Lime Juice

This is a really tasty way of making fruit salad known as Som Tum Pollamai *in Thailand. The Thai herbs make it very fresh, zesty, and quite different. You can use any fruits, but the ones I have chosen here are some of the most nutrient-rich of their type. Granny Smith apples have been found to contain up to 17 times more phytonutrients than other apple varieties. Dark-colored berries have increased amounts of anthocyanins, which are powerful antioxidants.*

Serves 4
1 **Granny Smith apple, unpeeled, halved, cored, and sliced into half moons**
2½ **cups dark berries (choose from blueberries, blackberries, strawberries, raspberries, or red grapes)**
2 **white-fleshed peaches or nectarines, sliced**
1 **mango, peeled and sliced or diced**
Seeds from ½ **pomegranate**

For the dressing:
3 **tablespoons raw honey or raw date syrup (see page 119)**
2 **tablespoons freshly squeezed lime juice**
¼ **teaspoon sea salt**
1 **tablespoon very finely chopped lemongrass**
8–10 **mint leaves, finely chopped**
Zest of 1 lime

To serve
Handful of shredded coconut, lightly toasted in the oven
Fresh yogurt (coconut yogurt would be very good if you can find it)

Put all the prepared fruit in a bowl. Combine the honey or date syrup, lime juice, and salt in another bowl. Stir, pour over the fruit, and toss well. Let the fruit sit for 5 minutes. Just before serving, add the chopped lemongrass, mint, and lime zest.

Scoop into bowls and top with coconut and yogurt. Eat when fresh.

SOUPS

&

SALADS

Here is a selection of dishes to get you through various seasons and moods. I have tried to keep the salads more of a side salad selection to go with the main dishes, but you could always beef them up by adding whatever is on hand as I often do. I am always improvising and making things up as I go along; sometimes it's the best way to discover something new. However, if it's a little inspiration you need or some seasonal guidance, then peek through this chapter for some delicious ideas. I tend to make my salad and soup recipes with flexibility in mind so that you could rustle them up for a lunch or a dinner, by adding other things. Sometimes there is nothing nicer than a simple radish salad with a beautiful piece of fresh soft cheese and a squeeze of lemon and some fresh herbs, lending their greenness and bite. With simple recipes, I wanted to show you how easy it is to whip up something healthy and really yummy too.

CHICKEN SOUP

For the Soul (two ways)

This soup is pretty much foolproof, and in terms of health benefits, it's liquid gold. Whenever my son or I feel poorly, I make a big batch and drink a cup of this broth morning, noon, and night. They don't call it Jewish penicillin for nothing! It really is the most restorative, healing, soothing, and nourishing thing you can drink. I have shown the two ways I make it most; both are tasty.

Makes 1 large pot serving 4–6
1 whole free-range organic chicken, rinsed
1 teaspoon black peppercorns
3 bay leaves
3 celery stalks, cut into chunks
2 onions, peeled and quartered
2 garlic cloves, peeled
4 carrots, cut into chunks
3 tablespoons unfiltered apple cider vinegar
Handful of parsley
A few sprigs of thyme
Hearty pinch or two of sea salt

To serve
Either
Bunch of purple or green curly kale, leaves stripped from stalks and chopped
Bunch of carrots, sliced thinly on the diagonal
Salt and pepper to taste
3¾–4 cups (roughly) cooked quinoa
Juice of 1 lemon
3 tablespoons raw coconut oil
A few sprigs of thyme
Or
Fresh ginger, peeled and finely grated
Salt and pepper to taste
Small bunch of mint
Small bunch of cilantro
1 medium chile, seeded and finely sliced
Juice of 1 lemon
3 tablespoons raw coconut oil

To make the broth, put everything for the soup into a really big stockpot and just cover it all with filtered water if possible; otherwise use tap water—the better the water the bigger the benefits.

Bring to a boil over high heat, reduce the heat to a very light simmer, only just bubbling, then place the lid on and simmer for 3 hours. Let the stock cool a bit and then strain. Discard all but the chicken.

Remove all the meat from the bones in lovely big chunks—don't shred it. Transfer the cooled stock back into the pot along with the chicken meat.

At this point you will have chosen which flavors you want to add from the serving options. If using kale and carrots, add them to the pot, simmer for 10 minutes, or until the carrots are tender, and taste for seasoning. Add the cooked quinoa to the pot and let it sit for a minute. Ladle the soup into bowls, squeeze a little lemon juice over each one together with ½ tablespoon of coconut oil, and top with a sprig of thyme. Or, if using ginger, cilantro, mint, and chile, simply add the grated ginger to the soup in the pot, reheat, taste for seasoning, then ladle into bowls. Add a few leaves of each herb into the bowls and top with a few slices of chile, a squeeze of lemon juice, and ½ tablespoon of coconut oil. Serve hot.

RUBY CHARD SOUP

This is a simple soup; it's a light, summery one and a great way of using greens. You can use any kind of chard or even kale if you can't get your hands on the ruby chard. The light vegetable or chicken broth is very restorative, while also being full of flavor.

Makes 1 large pot
3 tablespoons cold-pressed sunflower oil or raw odorless coconut oil
1 large yellow onion, finely diced
8 stems ruby chard, stalks removed and sliced and leaves cut into 1 in strips
2 × 14 oz cans cannellini beans, rinsed and drained
2½ quarts vegetable or chicken stock
5-6 tablespoons chili oil
Salt and pepper to taste

Heat the olive oil in a large pot over high heat and add the diced onion. Allow it to sizzle a bit, then turn the heat down to low and sauté for about 5–6 minutes until the onion is translucent; you don't want it to brown. Add the ruby chard, leaves, and stalks. Add the beans and then gently pour in the stock.

Simmer for about 20 minutes, remove from the heat, and taste for seasoning.

Serve in warmed bowls, drizzled with the chili oil.

BORLOTTI BEANS

with Artichoke Hearts

This little side is great with chicken, fish, or roasted vegetables. It goes spectacularly well with garlic aïoli and a piece of grilled white fish with herbs—a most heavenly combination.

Serves 4–6 as a side
10 roasted artichoke hearts in oil, with some of the oil
2 × 14 oz cans borlotti beans, rinsed and drained
Squeeze of lemon juice
Sea salt and freshly ground black pepper

Place a frying pan over high heat and, while it is warming, slice the artichoke hearts into quarters and throw them into the pan along with a couple of tablespoons of the oil from the jar.

Add the beans and stir them carefully—you want the beans to stay as whole as possible. Cook them only as long as it takes for them to be warmed through—this will take 2–3 minutes.

Spoon them into a serving bowl, squeeze over a little lemon juice, and sprinkle with a little sea salt and freshly ground black pepper.

RADISH SALAD

with Lemon & Parsley

For such a small vegetable, radishes really pack a serious punch in the health department. For a start, they cleanse the body and help it to eliminate toxins and free radicals, they soothe the digestive system, prevent viral infections, and keep you hydrated.

Serves 4 as a side
1¼ lbs round radishes (the colorful ones are
   pretty if you can find them)
Juice of ½ lemon
Olive oil
Sea salt and freshly ground black pepper
Small handful of parsley, finely sliced

Simply slice all the radishes into thin little rounds and place them into a serving bowl. Squeeze over some lemon juice, drizzle with a little oil, and season with salt and pepper. Lastly, scatter with the parsley, give everything a good toss, and serve.

PUY LENTILS

with Wilted Spinach

A delicious grain-free side—earthy, protein-rich lentils are sublime cooked with silky, buttery, wilted spinach. Great with Roast Pumpkin, Golden Beet, and Squash Salad (see page 59) and Hummus (see page 107), or maybe a piece of fish or chicken and some homemade Mayonnaise (see page 111).

Serves 4
1 cup puy lentils
3 cups chicken or vegetable stock or water
A few teaspoons of olive oil
Pat of butter
3 cups baby spinach
Sea salt and freshly ground black pepper

Rinse the lentils under running water and then put them into a large pot and cover with stock or water. Bring to a boil and simmer for 20–25 minutes—you want them with a bit of a bite, not mushy. Drain.

Put a large frying pan over medium–high heat and add the drained lentils, oil, and butter. Throw in your spinach and cook until just wilting—it will only take a minute. Season to taste and serve.

FENNEL SALAD

with Blood Oranges, Buffalo Mozzarella & Dill

This has to be one for special occasions, as blood oranges are only available for a short time. They are a joy to behold, and make a delicious pairing with the mozzarella, dill, and fennel. This salad is cleansing and has a bright clean taste—I love it with roast chicken and a big green salad. It's delicious as a topping for a slice of toasted sourdough rye bread that has had a light rub with a garlic clove and a drizzle of oil... so very good! Great for lunch or a merry get together as part of a dinner.

Serves 6
2 fennel bulbs, trimmed
2 blood oranges, peeled to remove any of the
  outer white pith and membrane (use ordinary
  oranges when blood oranges are out of season)
2 balls of buffalo mozzarella
4 sprigs of dill, leaves picked
¼ cup really good cold-pressed olive oil
Juice of ½ lemon
Sea salt and freshly cracked pepper

Start by taking a very thin slice off the very bottom of the fennel. This removes any brown bits and gives a nice flat base so that you can set the fennel upright to slice it. Now slice the fennel as thinly as you can.

Arrange the fennel and orange slices on a shallow serving platter. Tear up the mozzarella into medium pieces and arrange over the orange and fennel. Scatter with the dill, then drizzle with the olive oil and squeeze over the juice from the lemon. Add a pinch of sea salt and a few twists of pepper. Enjoy.

MY SMASHED CUCUMBER SALAD

This is a great way of using up an abundance of cucumbers, which can easily happen in the summertime. It is a delightful little salad, fresh and zingy, to accompany a barbecue if you're cooking meat or chicken. It's super cleansing and the enzymes, herbs, and ginger help to digest richer food on the menu.

Serves 6
For the dressing:
1 garlic clove, finely grated
2 in piece of fresh ginger, peeled and finely grated
3 tablespoons apple cider vinegar
1½ teaspoons maple syrup
2 teaspoons toasted sesame oil
Pinch of sea salt

3 cucumbers, peeled
2 scallions, sliced into thin rounds
½ green chile, seeded and finely sliced
½ red chile, seeded and finely sliced
5 teaspoons finely chopped mint leaves (or shiso leaves if you can find them)
4 teaspoons finely chopped cilantro leaves
Sea salt and freshly ground black pepper

To make the dressing, combine the garlic, ginger, vinegar, syrup, and oil. Give it a good whisk and then add a pinch of salt.

Cut the cucumbers into 2½ in chunks and then crush them using the flat blade of a large knife. Throw them into a bowl, add the scallions, chiles, mint and cilantro leaves, a pinch of salt, and a few twists of pepper. Add the dressing, toss well and serve.

PARSNIPS *with* PARMESAN HASH

This is true comfort food, which is quick and really easy to make. It's also a different way of using parsnips; they're almost more delicious done this way than roasted. Great with an egg for breakfast or as a side for lunch or dinner.

Serves 4
3 tablespoons extra virgin olive oil
2 medium floury potatoes, scrubbed clean, halved lengthwise, and thinly sliced into half moons
2 parsnips, peeled, halved lengthwise, and thinly sliced into half moons
1 small onion, finely minced
½ cup shaved Parmesan cheese
Sea salt and freshly ground black pepper

Preheat a large nonstick pan over medium–high heat and add the oil. Add the potatoes and parsnips with a little seasoning and stir for 10–12 minutes or until the vegetables are cooked through and nicely colored. Add the onion and continue cooking until everything is golden.

Remove from the heat and stir in the cheese. Taste for seasoning and serve.

ROAST FENNEL

with Cherry Tomatoes

My rule for cooking fennel is, if it's to be eaten raw, slice it as thinly as possible and, if you're cooking it, do it gently with lots of butter and good oils. Also, fennel LOVES lemon, so add lots of zest whether you're serving it raw or cooked. This is perfect as a bed for a little roasted sea bass or it would go beautifully with some Quinoa (see page 62) and garlicky Mayonnaise (see page 111). Heaven.

Serves 6
3 fennel bulbs
1½ tablespoons butter (or if you don't want to use butter just use extra oil)
Zest and juice of ½ lemon
A few good teaspoons of olive oil
1¼ cups cherry tomatoes, preferably on the vine
Sea salt and freshly ground black pepper

Preheat the oven to 350°F. Trim the bases off your fennel and tidy up the tops, removing any feathery leaves that don't look good to eat. Slice the fennel lengthwise into wedges—depending on the size of the bulb, I usually cut each half into 3 wedges. Lay the wedges in a baking dish, dot a few pieces of butter (if using) over the top, sprinkle with the zest, and drizzle with oil.

Transfer to the oven and bake for 25 minutes. Place the cherry tomatoes on top of the cooking fennel and put the dish back in the oven for another 15 minutes, or until the tomatoes are starting to collapse and the skins are deliciously split with a bit of color.

Squeeze over the lemon juice, sprinkle with a little salt and pepper, and serve.

MY FAVORITE MASHED ROOT VEGETABLES

This is my favorite mash. I totally prefer it to mashed potatoes, which I find can be a bit boring. And I'm pretty sure once you've tried this colorful version you won't want conventional mashed potatoes either! It's earthy, creamy, nourishing, and delicious—and it goes with pretty much anything. Top with snipped chives.

Serves 4
1 cup parsnips, peeled and cut into chunks
2 cups sweet potato, peeled and cut into chunks
3 cups butternut squash, peeled and cut into chunks
½ cup milk
Bay leaf
½ teaspoon finely grated or ground nutmeg
3½ tablespoons butter
Sea salt and freshly ground black pepper
3 tablespoons coarsely chopped chives

Keep the parsnips separate from the sweet potato and squash. Put the parsnips in a small saucepan with the milk, bay leaf, and nutmeg and cook until tender. Put the sweet potato and butternut squash in a second pan of salted water and cook until tender.

Drain all the vegetables, reserving the milk from the parsnips. Spread the vegetables onto a flat pan, again keeping the parsnips separate, and allow everything to dry off for a couple of minutes.

Transfer the parsnips to a bowl and process with an immersion blender. Add a pat of the butter and enough milk to give a smooth finish. Warm the remaining milk and butter in the saucepan you used to cook the vegetables, add the potato and squash, then mash in the pan, off the heat, until smooth. Add the parsnips and stir well. Scoop into a serving bowl and sprinkle with chives.

ROAST PUMPKIN, GOLDEN BEET & SQUASH SALAD

with Garlic

This warm salad is seriously nourishing, and the combination of silky squash, earthy beets, and the potent garlic make a flavorful dish that you will love. It's colorful and super easy to make. It's great with some Hummus (see page 107) and greens for lunch or as a side to something more substantial for dinner.

Serves 8

½ **butternut squash, halved lengthwise, seeds removed**

4 **golden beets, peeled and cut into 6 wedges**

1 **medium orange pumpkin (acorn squash or Japanese red kuri), halved, seeds removed**

1 **whole bulb garlic, cloves separated and unpeeled**

A few tablespoons of olive oil

Sea salt and freshly ground pepper

Preheat the oven to 350°F. Slice the butternut squash into four long slices and place on a big baking sheet with the golden beet wedges. Cut the pumpkin halves into lovely crescent moon wedges—roughly four wedges per half pumpkin—and scatter those on the pan too with the garlic cloves.

Drizzle olive oil generously over everything, sprinkle with sea salt and pepper, and roast in the oven for about 30–35 minutes. Keep an eye on them; you want the edges to start browning and the vegetables to be tender all the way through—check by inserting a small sharp knife into a thick piece.

Remove the vegetables from the oven and let cool a little. Transfer everything to a shallow platter and serve.

KALE

with Lemon & Caramelized Red Onions

You could also try this with cavolo nero, if you can find it. Apart from tasting amazing, both curly kale and cavolo nero are full of vitamins K and A as well as significant amounts of magnesium, copper, fiber, calcium, iron, and B vitamins. They're incredibly restorative and nourishing and a great source of fiber. Being cooked with sweet onions and sharpened with a squeeze of lemon at the end bring it all to life.

Serves 4

10–12 stems kale (or you can use cavolo nero)
Big pat of butter, or 1 tablespoon odorless raw coconut oil
Generous drizzle of olive oil
1 large red onion, halved and sliced into thin half moons
Sea salt and freshly ground black pepper
Juice of ½ lemon

Put a large frying pan with a lid over high heat. While it's warming, give the kale or cavolo nero a quick rinse and then strip the central stalks away from the leafy green bits. Discard the tough stalks.

Put the butter and olive oil into the hot pan and, when it sizzles, add the onion and turn down the heat to medium–low, stirring the onions all the time—you don't want them to stick. After 8 minutes they should be soft and sweet.

Throw in the kale or cavolo nero and a tablespoon or two of water—just enough to steam the vegetables a little—and cover with the lid; the water will evaporate as the leaves cook, provided you don't add too much.

A couple of minutes later, lift the lid and stir. You may need to turn up the heat again if it's not bubbling and steaming: keep an eye on it. It needs to cook for about 4–5 minutes. If the pan dries out too much, add a small pat of butter.

When everything is lovely and cooked and smelling delicious, take the pan off the heat, add a sprinkle of salt and a few twists of pepper, then squeeze over your lemon. Serve.

STEAMED VEGETABLES

Japanese Style

*If ever I feel I have slightly overindulged, this is the perfect antidote, a simple and clean
way to enjoy produce at its best. You could serve these vegetables as an accompaniment,
but I often prefer to have them just as they are. It's especially satisfying if you are able to
pick the vegetables straight from the garden, sun-warmed and full of goodness.*

Serves 2–4
**An assortment of seasonal vegetables, e.g.
pumpkins or squash, sweet potatoes (peeled),
carrots, cauliflower, broccoli, green beans,
sugar snap peas, asparagus**
Flaky sea salt
Good quality olive oil
½ lemon

For the dipping sauce:
¼ cup good quality soy sauce
2 tablespoons mirin
1½ in piece of fresh ginger, peeled and finely grated
2 teaspoons maple syrup
½ teaspoon toasted sesame oil

To serve
Small handful of chopped scallions
2 tablespoons lightly toasted sunflower seeds
2 tablespoons lightly toasted pumpkin seeds
2 tablespoons lightly toasted sesame seeds

Equipment
**1 steamer or a 3-tiered bamboo steamer
that will fit inside a large pot with a lid**

Once you have chosen your vegetables, cut them into bite-sized pieces that are on the large side. Arrange them in a single layer with the vegetables that take longest to cook, for example the pumpkin or squash and sweet potato together in one basket, broccoli, cauliflower, and carrots in another, and quicker-cooking ones like beans and peas in the top basket.

Put your steamer or large pot, with a couple of inches of water in the bottom, over high heat and bring it to a boil. Don't add too much water or it will rise up through the base of the steamer and boil the vegetables instead of steaming them.

Place your basket with the vegetables that take longest to cook in first. Put the lid on and leave them to steam for about 6–7 minutes, by which time they will be about two-thirds cooked. Now place the second tier in position, cover, and steam for another 3–4 minutes. Finally, place the top tier in position, cover again, and steam for 1 minute—this way all the vegetables should be ready at the same time: bright yet tender and steamed through. Check by inserting a small sharp knife into the vegetables—it should slide through easily.

Arrange all the vegetables on a single plate or serving tray. Sprinkle with the scallions and toasted seeds if you wish and take to the table just as it is. Mix together the ingredients for the dipping sauce in a small bowl and serve with the vegetables.

QUINOA

with a Rainbow of Jewels

I first made this for my friend Ieva on her birthday. It's a beautiful way to present quinoa, the tiny grains and pomegranate seeds really do look like jewels and it's packed with delicious flavors. You can also use this as a base for a hearty stew or casserole, or serve for lunch with some avocado and a green leaf salad.

Serves 6–8
3 small red onions
Good olive oil
Sea salt and freshly ground black pepper
½ butternut squash, peeled and cut into
    ½ in squares
3¾–4 cups cooked quinoa at room temperature
Seeds from 1 pomegranate
1¼ cups parsley, finely chopped
¾ cup mint, leaves picked and finely chopped
Juice of 1 lemon

To serve
A few fronds of dill, leaves picked
Rose petals, washed (must be unsprayed),
    (optional)

Preheat the oven to 350°F. Cut the onions in half from top to bottom then peel them, leaving the base intact (you may want to trim off the top though). Cut each half into three wedges—the base will hold the slices together. Put them on a small baking sheet, drizzle with olive oil, and sprinkle with salt and pepper. Transfer the pan to the oven.

Do the same with the squash on a second baking sheet. Keep an eye on them both: after about 15–20 minutes, the red onion should be tender and a little caramelized around the edges. As soon as it's ready, remove the pan. The squash will need another 10–15 minutes before it's tender and a little colored at the edges.

When both vegetables are cooked, put the quinoa in a big serving bowl. Lay the squash and red onion on top, scatter with two-thirds of the pomegranate seeds, the parsley, mint, and the lemon juice. Drizzle with a generous amount of olive oil. Sprinkle in a good few pinches of sea salt and a few twists of pepper. Using two big spoons, gently toss to mix.

Serve sprinkled with the remaining pomegranate seeds, the dill leaves, and rose petals (if using).

MAIN DISHES

I have based this chapter around ingredients I like to eat for my evening meals—dishes that can be added to or eaten as they are on their own with a simple green salad on the side. There is a cross section—from a simple vegetable chili to a sumptuous Mexican Feast. All are super healthy and full of goodness, with immune-boosting qualities and good fats. The main mealtime of the day for me is dinner. I was brought up in a big family and we always sat down to eat together. This is something I have carried on in my own family with my son. As long as I am not working, I will always eat with him. This encourages healthy and positive eating habits and it is a great way to sit and share the day. Sometimes I have the energy to go all out, so to speak, and other nights dinner can be as simple as an omelet with a green salad. As long as it has some healthy fats and plenty of fiber, even a frugal supper can be incredibly nourishing. My taste buds tend to take me around the world and my son loves nothing more than a beautiful curry, freshly made with all good things or the indulgent Mexican Feast. For this reason I wanted to include some different bold flavors from around the world, things I cook regularly when I am busy or when I have more time. Either way you will find good nourishment for your body.

MY NOURISH BOWL

The idea behind a Nourish Bowl is to have something that nourishes all aspects of the self: taste, nutrition, and something that nourishes visually. It's about choosing nutrient-dense vegetables, healthy fats, quality proteins, and some probiotic foods to make a filling meal in a bowl.
It's a great thing to have as a lunch in particular, but could easily work for a delicious dinner. It's endlessly versatile and can be varied to suit what you like or what you have in the garden or fridge.
This is more of a guide than a recipe. Here, I show how I might put together my Nourish Bowl, but you can add whatever you like. There are some good things to choose from in the Sides and Main Dishes chapter of this book, so you can build the rest of your Nourish Bowl around things you already have recipes for. For example, if you have a recipe for hummus and you have some chicken or tempeh, that's great: just add some healthy fats and some nutrient-dense vegetables et voilà!
Whichever ingredients you choose, it should be simple and fun to make, a bit like throwing a beautiful salad together.

For the protein:
Tempeh
Fish
Turkey
Chicken
Eggs, softly boiled with
 runny yolks
Vegetable chili (see page 79)
Cheeses
Lentils
Hummus (see page 107)
Tamari seeds / toasted seeds
Nuts
Quinoa

For the good fats:
Avocado / Guacamole
 (see page 72)
Cheese
Cold-pressed oils
 (see page 247)
Nuts / seeds

Raw and cooked nutrient-dense veggies:
Beets
Red rose sprouts/ any sprout
Radishes
Globe artichokes
Roast or steamed pumpkin
Tomatoes
Green beans
Bitter leaves / arugula / watercress /
 dandelion / raddichio / mizuna

Probiotic foods:
Sauerkraut
Kimchi (see page 110)
Lacto-fermented veg
 i.e., radishes, cauliflower, carrots

Arrange what you have chosen and prepared around the bowl. Drizzle with lemon juice and really good quality extra virgin olive oil, and sprinkle with good quality sea salt and freshly cracked black pepper.

JAPANESE BROWN RICE BOWL

& Kimchi, two ways

For the protein add either fish or tempeh, a fermented, cooked soy bean product from Indonesia that has more protein and fiber than the more familiar tofu. Brown rice and quinoa are both fantastic for the fiber and micronutrients they provide.

Serves 6–8
3½–4 cups cooked brown rice or quinoa

For the roasted vegetables:
1 medium pumpkin or butternut squash, halved, seeds removed and sliced into long wedges
Knob of fresh ginger, peeled and grated
1 garlic clove, finely grated
2 teaspoons toasted sesame oil
2 tablespoons tamari, shoyu, or other good quality soy sauce
2 tablespoons cold-pressed sunflower oil

For the caramelized sprouts:
1 lb Brussels sprouts, trimmed (or other green vegetables e.g. beans or broccoli)
3–4 tablespoons cold-pressed sunflower oil
Sea salt and pepper to taste

For the protein:
Vegetarian: 1 pack of tempeh, cut into 1 in slices and added to the pumpkin when roasting
Fish: 12 small sardines or 4 medium mackerel, cleaned
Olive oil
Juice of ½ lemon
Sea salt and freshly ground black pepper

To serve
2 teaspoons furikake or 2 teaspoons toasted black or white sesame seeds
Extra tamari for drizzling on the rice or quinoa
Small bowl of Kimchi (see page 110)
1 lemon, cut into wedges

Preheat the oven to 350°F. Put the pumpkin or squash in a roasting pan and toss with the other ingredients. If you're following the vegetarian option, add your tempeh to the pan too. Roast for 30 minutes or until the pumpkin is tender right through and starting to brown at the edges.

Meanwhile, caramelize your Brussels sprouts: Half fill a medium saucepan with boiling water, place over high heat, drop in the sprouts, and blanch for about 2 minutes. Remove from the heat and plunge into cold water. Drain then dry the sprouts and cut each one in half.

Set a frying pan over relatively high heat, add the oil, and toss in the sprouts. Cook, stirring every so often, until lovely and caramelized (6–8 minutes). Do keep an eye on them as the sugars in the sprouts mean they can burn easily. Once cooked, remove from the heat and set aside to keep warm.

If you are adding fish to your meal, preheat a grill pan until smoking hot. Wash the sardines or mackerel, dry them with paper towels, toss in a little oil, and place on the hot grill pan. Cook on both sides until charred; this should take 2–3 minutes on each side for sardines and 5–6 minutes for mackerel; you can always finish them in the oven if it's easier and less smoky. Remove from the heat, squeeze over the lemon juice, and season with a little salt and pepper.

To serve, place the different components into serving bowls and allow people to help themselves.

JAPANESE CHICKEN

This is super and you can also make it using fillets of white fish or salmon as well—just don't cook for so long. It's AMAZING with My Smashed Cucumber Salad (see page 56) and roast pumpkin, brown rice, or quinoa—or beet quinoa for a very colorful plate.

Serves 4–6
8–10 chicken thighs, bone in, skin removed

For the marinade:
4 fat garlic cloves, finely grated
1½ in piece of fresh ginger, peeled and finely grated
2 teaspoons fermented brown miso
3 tablespoons dark honey
3 tablespoons naturally fermented tamari
½ teaspoon chile powder (if you can find it, togarashi is amazing—omit if feeding children)

To serve
Smashed Cucumber Salad (see page 56)

Wash and dry the chicken thighs. Mix all the marinade ingredients in a large bowl.

Add the chicken and toss the pieces really well to make sure they are well-coated. Cover and place in the fridge for several hours or overnight.

Preheat the oven to 350°F. Place the chicken pieces in a shallow roasting dish, so that the pieces fit in a single layer quite snugly. Pour in the sauce. Transfer the dish to the oven and roast for 50 minutes, basting every now and then.

Meanwhile, prepare the Smashed Cucumber Salad.

The chicken is cooked when the juices run clear when poked with the tip of a sharp knife and the meat is starting to fall off the bone.

Serve with brown rice or quinoa.

LEMON & SUMAC CHICKEN

with Cherry Tomatoes & Black Olives

This is easy to throw together but it's still full of flavor and color. My favorite kind of meal... It would be good with Fennel Salad with Blood Oranges (see page 54) for a light summery lunch or dinner or with Roast Pumpkin, Golden Beet & Squash Salad (see page 59), for a more nourishing winter meal. Kids and adults both love this and it's a firm favorite in my household.

Serves 4–6
4 free-range whole chicken legs
Handful of good quality black olives
Olive oil
2 teaspoons sumac
Large handful of sweet ripe cherry tomatoes
1 preserved lemon, sliced into thin rounds (available in specialty grocery stores)
Sea salt and freshly cracked or ground black pepper

Preheat the oven to 350°F. Wash and dry the chicken pieces and place in a roasting dish. Scatter the black olives on top and drizzle with olive oil. Sprinkle with the sumac and some salt and black pepper.

Transfer the dish to the middle rack of the oven and cook for 30 minutes. Top with the cherry tomatoes and lemon slices, then cook for another 20–30 minutes—you want the tomatoes bursting, the lemons a little charred, and the meat falling off the bone.

Serve while hot and fresh from the oven. I love to eat this chicken dish with a beautiful, bitter raddichio salad.

MEXICAN FEAST

Mexican Feast serves 4–6

To serve
2 packs of fresh corn tortillas
¾ cup sour cream

Prepare the chicken first then, while it's marinating, prepare the other recipes. When you are ready to eat, toast your corn tortillas in a hot pan, allowing 30 seconds per side, then pile them onto a plate and cover with a kitchen towel as you go to keep them warm.

Simply lay everything out on the table and make up tortillas with different combinations each time as and how you like. Serve with the corn alongside and top your tortillas with either sour cream or slices of pickled red onion or both! Enjoy.

REFRIED BEANS WITH FETA

Olive oil
1 large onion, finely diced
1 garlic clove, finely chopped
1 × 14 oz can black pinto beans and their liquid
1 teaspoon chipotle chile powder, plus a little extra
Sea salt and freshly ground black pepper
¾ cup feta

Heat a little oil in a medium saucepan, add the onion, and sauté for about 5 minutes, then add the garlic and beans, liquid and all. Simmer gently for about 20 minutes. Add the chipotle powder and simmer for another 5 minutes. If the beans are getting too dry, add a little water, as they will thicken up as they cool—don't make them too runny, though. Remove from the heat, scoop into a bowl, and crumble in the feta. Sprinkle with a little extra chipotle powder.

GUACAMOLE

6 ripe avocados, halved, pits removed
Zest and juice of 1 lemon
2 limes, zest of 1 and juice of both
1 medium red onion, finely diced
2 garlic cloves, finely grated
Small bunch of cilantro, coarsely chopped, plus extra sprigs to serve
8 tablespoons cold-pressed olive oil, plus extra to drizzle
Sea salt and freshly ground black pepper

Scoop the flesh of the avocados into a medium bowl and mash with a fork. Squeeze over the lemon and lime juice, mix, then add all the other ingredients. Check the seasoning, adding a little salt and pepper to taste. Transfer to a serving bowl, drizzle with a little olive oil, and garnish with a few sprigs of cilantro.

GRILLED CORN ON THE COB WITH SMOKED PAPRIKA & SALT

4 corn on the cob, husks removed and each cob cut into 3
2 tablespoons cold-pressed sunflower oil
1 teaspoon sea salt and a few twists of black pepper
1 teaspoon smoked paprika

Bring a medium pan of water to a boil, drop in the corn, and simmer gently with the lid on for about 10 minutes; drain, dry, and set aside.

Bring a grill pan to smoking point. While the pan is heating, drizzle the oil over the corn and then place them carefully onto the hot pan, moving every now and then to char on all sides—this should take 2–3 minutes.

Remove from the pan and sprinkle with the salt and smoked paprika. Pile the corn high onto a beautiful plate.

PICKLED RED ONIONS

2 teaspoons black peppercorns
8 whole allspice berries
2 cloves
1 level teaspoon oregano
1 medium red onion, halved
  and sliced into thin half moons
¾ teaspoon sea salt
¼ cup apple cider vinegar
3 juicy limes, squeezed

First grind the peppercorns, allspice, cloves, and oregano to a coarse powder using a mortar and pestle or a spice grinder.

Put the sliced onion into a medium bowl, add the spice mix and massage it into the onion, then add salt, vinegar, and lime juice. Mix everything really well.

Transfer the mix to a tall sterilized narrow jar with a tight-fitting lid. Let it marinate for 24 hours, giving the jar an occasional shake before using. These pickled onions will keep in the fridge for up to a week.

PICO DE GALLO

2 cups cherry tomatoes
1 medium red chile, finely diced
1 medium green chile, finely diced
1 small red onion, finely diced
1 garlic clove, finely grated
Juice of 1 lime
Zest and juice of ½ lemon
Small bunch of cilantro,
  coarsely chopped

Chop all the tomatoes into small pieces—either into halves or quarters, depending on size. Put them in a bowl along with all the other ingredients and mix thoroughly. Transfer to a serving bowl and keep cool until ready to use.

MY MEXICAN FRESH SALAD

1 red onion, halved lengthwise and
  sliced into thin half moons
1 cucumber, cut into finger-size
  pieces
Bunch of cilantro
2 limes, each cut into 8 wedges

Arrange all the ingredients on a beautiful plate.

SHREDDED CHICKEN THIGHS MARINATED WITH GINGER & CHILE

8 chicken thighs, skins removed
4 dried guajillo chiles, wiped
  clean, de-stemmed, slit open,
  seeded, and deveined
¾ in piece of fresh ginger, peeled
2 garlic cloves
1 teaspoon ground cumin
1½ teaspoons salt
½ cup cold-pressed olive oil

Place the chicken thighs in a large bowl. Soak the dried chiles in warm water for 30 minutes. Drain and put in a food processor with the ginger, garlic, cumin, salt, and olive oil. Add ½ cup of water and process until smooth. Pour the marinade over the chicken and massage gently. Cover the bowl for at least 4 hours or overnight to marinate.

Preheat the oven to 350°F. Transfer the chicken and all the marinade into an ovenproof dish and roast gently for about 1 hour, or until the meat starts to fall off the bone.

Remove from the oven and carefully shred all the chicken off the bone in large flakes using two forks. Place the shredded chicken into a lovely serving bowl for the feast.

A PERFECTLY COOKED PIECE OF FISH

Serves 1

1 fillet of fish with skin on or off, roughly 8 oz per person (e.g. salmon, sea bass, haddock, cod, snapper)
Sea salt and black pepper
Olive oil, ghee, or grapeseed oil
A pat of butter
½ lemon

Place a heavy-bottomed steel pan over medium–high heat for several minutes until very hot. A nonstick pan won't get the skin really brown and golden.

First wash the fillet, then dry it well with a paper towel to make the skin crisp. Season both sides with sea salt and pepper.

Coat a hot pan with a little oil, something with a high smoke point like ghee or grapeseed is great. Allow the oil to heat and, when it starts to smoke, quickly add your fish, skin-side down. The proteins will immediately react and the fillet will contract and curve upward. Take a flexible spatula and press the entire fillet gently back down and hold for a few seconds to ensure even cooking and crispy skin all over.

Flip near the end of cooking. Let the fish cook; don't mess with it too much, just let it go. When you can see a lovely golden brown color on the edge of the skin, and the edges of the fish are turning an opaque color, carefully and gently use a spatula to life up the fillet and turn it over. The fish is delicate, so flip it carefully so it doesn't all break up. At this point it's about 70 percent cooked, so it will only need another couple of minutes on the other side.

You can add a pat of butter at this point for flavor if you like and baste the fish while it finishes cooking. Remove from the pan and serve.

BAKED HADDOCK

with Ginger, Tomatoes & Pine Nuts

This is one of those wonderful recipes that looks great, tastes amazing, and yet is so easy to make. It's great with a big green salad, or Puy Lentils with Wilted Spinach (see page 53). It's a great summery dish.

Serves 4
4 medium fillets of haddock (roughly 6 oz each)

For the marinade:
Small handful of basil leaves, torn
1 medium red chile, seeded and finely sliced
3 tablespoons olive oil
Generous handful of cherry tomatoes
Generous pinch of sea salt flakes
2 tablespoons lemon juice
2 tablespoons water
¾ in piece of fresh ginger, peeled and finely grated
1 garlic clove, finely grated
1 cups pine nuts

To serve
10 mint leaves, torn
½ red chile, seeded and sliced
Small handful of basil leaves, torn

Put the fish fillets in a roasting dish just big enough to hold them comfortably without being too cramped.

Mix the ingredients for the marinade and rub over the fillets, cover, and let marinate for 1 hour.

Preheat the oven to 350°F. Transfer the marinated fish to the middle rack of the oven and cook for 12–15 minutes, depending on the size of the fillets. Once cooked, remove from the oven and allow to sit for another 2 minutes.

Sprinkle with torn mint leaves, extra chile, and basil. Serve immediately.

SEAFOOD & FENNEL STEW

with Tarragon Gremolata

This is a winning combination of Mediterranean flavors—seafood, fennel, tomatoes, garlic, and preserved lemon—and the Tarragon Gremolata (see page 106) really makes the dish sing. I will happily eat this stew on its own, but it would also be rather good served on a bed of quinoa.

Serves 6
Good drizzle olive oil
3 large garlic cloves, finely sliced
3 fennel bulbs, trimmed and cut into wedges,
   fronds reserved for garnish
2¾ cups fish stock
½ medium preserved lemon, quartered
8 large vine tomatoes, quartered
1 tablespoon sweet paprika
Good pinch of saffron
Small handful of chopped flat-leaf parsley
2 fillets of salmon, (9 oz) skin removed, cut into thirds
2 fillets of cod or other white fish, (9 oz) skin
   removed, cut into thirds
12 mussels
24 clams
6 jumbo shrimp
Sea salt and freshly ground black pepper

To serve
Tarragon Gremolata (see page 106)

Put the olive oil and garlic in a large, heavy-bottomed pan or stockpot and cook over medium–low heat for 2 minutes. Add the fennel wedges and cook for another 3–4 minutes.

Stir in the stock and the preserved lemon, bring to a boil, and then cover and reduce the heat to a gentle simmer. Cook for 10 minutes. Add the tomatoes, spices, and the parsley. Cook for another 5 minutes.

Add the pieces of fish, the seafood, and up to ¾ cup water—enough to ensure the liquid in the pan covers the fish.

Put a lid on the pan and turn up the heat to a rolling boil. Cook for 3–4 minutes, or until the shellfish has opened and the shrimp is pink.

Using a slotted spoon, remove the shellfish and fish from the stew and continue to cook, uncovered, for 4–5 minutes until the liquid has reduced and slightly thickened. Discard any mussels or clams that remain closed.

Taste for seasoning and add salt and pepper if required. Return the shellfish and fish to the pan for a minute or two. Serve hot, sprinkled with the Tarragon Gremolata.

My mother's

VEGETABLE CHILI

This is a super easy chili that lasts really well. It's packed full of protein and flavor. Kids love it, as do adults. I like to make big batches and keep it in the fridge, so it's easy to throw together a great dinner or lunch in 5 minutes. It's perfect after a strenuous day or a long exercise session. My favorite way of eating it is with crème fraîche and cilantro.

Serves 4–6

4 garlic cloves

¼ cup cold-pressed sunflower oil, raw coconut oil, or ghee

1 large yellow onion, finely diced

1 large carrot, cut into ½ in dice

1 red bell pepper, halved, seeded, and ribs removed, cut into ½ in dice

½ teaspoon mild chile powder

1 teaspoon cumin

Hearty pinch of sea salt and plenty of freshly cracked or ground black pepper

2 teaspoons chipotle in adobo sauce (or chipotle powder can be used)

3¼ cups tomato sauce (preferably from a glass jar)

½ cup puy lentils, rinsed

1 × 14 oz can black beans, rinsed and drained (or 2 cups fresh black beans after soaking and cooking)

1 × 14 oz can kidney beans, rinsed and drained (or 2 cups fresh kidney beans after soaking and cooking)

¼ cup tomato sauce

Small bunch of cilantro, finely chopped

To serve

Sour cream or crème fraîche

Cilantro leaves

Chile powder or extra chipotle

Start by mincing or chopping your garlic really finely and allow it to sit for 10 minutes while you prepare the rest of the vegetables.

Heat the oil or ghee in a large saucepan or stockpot over high heat. Add the onion, carrot, bell pepper, garlic, chile powder, and cumin, along with a hearty pinch of salt. When everything is hot and cooking nicely, turn the heat down a little and continue to sweat all the vegetables for about 10–15 minutes. You want them softened, sweet, and not coloring too much. After 15 minutes, stir in the chipotle.

At this point, turn the heat back up, add the tomato sauce (or homemade bottled tomatoes as my mother would), and be sure to pour in all the juices too. Bring to a boil. Reduce the heat and allow the vegetables to simmer for 25 minutes.

Throw in your rinsed lentils and beans and add one can of water to the pot, along with the tomato paste. Bring to a boil, reduce the heat, and simmer for 1 hour 20 minutes, adding a touch more water if it dries out too much. After it's cooked, let settle and cool a bit. Serve while hot with some sour cream or crème fraîche and cilantro.

SPRING ZUCCHINI "SPAGHETTI"

with Kale Pesto & Arugula Flowers

Making spaghetti from zucchini couldn't be easier, but you do need a spiralizer or special peeler—they are easy to find online or in kitchen stores. I have teamed my "spaghetti" here with spring peas, kale pesto, and arugula flowers. The arugula flowers are spicy and nutty; if you can't find the flowers you can just use arugula leaves. This is really light and delicious, yet a very nutrient-dense dish that will certainly give you a spring in your step. Since this dish is raw, it's great for late spring or early summer when lighter and more refreshing meals are the order of the day.

Serves 2
2 zucchini, spiralized

For the kale pesto:
½ cup cashews, lightly toasted
¾ cup parmesan, coarsely grated
3 garlic cloves
⅓ cup extra virgin olive oil
1¼ cups kale, leafy part only, not the inner stalk
A good squeeze of lemon
Sea salt and freshly cracked black pepper

To serve
Big drizzle cold-pressed extra virgin olive oil
Basil leaves, torn
Mint leaves, torn
A handful of freshly podded peas or lightly blanched frozen peas
Arugula flowers or a handful of arugula leaves
Shavings of Parmesean

Place everything for the pesto into a blender and pulse until you have a rough sauce, adding a little bit more lemon juice or Parmesan to taste if it needs more balance. Season to taste with salt and pepper

Place your zucchini spirals into a big serving bowl, top with just enough of the kale pesto to coat the noodles, reserving the rest for another occasion, then drizzle with the olive oil and give it a thorough but gentle stir. Strew with torn basil leaves, mint leaves, peas, arugula flowers or leaves, shavings of Parmesean, and a few twists of pepper.

SWEET TOOTH

As you may know, I have a bit of a sweet tooth. My last book was a healthy baking book and I have included in this chapter some more delightful things that happen in my kitchen on a regular basis. Everything from a three-layered celebration cake to healthy ice cream, decadent but super nourishing and totally good for you.

There are also some great snack ideas for those moments when we need a little pick up, when reserves are low. If you're like me and need to keep your energy levels up, and find it hard to make wise choices when sugar levels are low, then it's not fair to rely on will-power alone.

I would strongly recommend having a few things on hand in jars ready to eat when you need a quick pick-me-up. I always have soaked almonds in the fridge and a jar of grain-free granola on my shelf; it's perfect as a little snack.

My son loves ice cream, so I have come up with healthy ideas for ice creams that adults love too. Always have some frozen bananas and berries in your freezer ready to go. Then you can build on those flavors with other things that are in season or in your pantry. I am sure you will find plenty of inspiration in these next few pages for healthy snacks and treats.

CHIA PUDDING

with Apple Compôte, Fresh Raspberries, and Pistachios

This pudding is full of flavor, with healthy fats and omega oils from the chia seeds and milk. Healthy fats help to stabilize metabolism. Chia pudding is so easy to make and hits the spot when you need a bit of a treat. I love to make extra chia pudding to keep in the fridge so that I can add some fresh fruit and coconut yogurt whenever I need a little pick-me-up or for my son's afternoon snack. It will keep well there for up to a week.

Serves 2

1½ cups of your favorite milk, heated
¼ cup chia seeds
1 large Macintosh apple,
  peeled, cored, and cut into
  1¼ in pieces
1–2 teaspoons raw honey
  or raw date syrup (see page 119)
Seeds from ¼ vanilla bean
½ cup pistachios, chopped
Borage flowers (optional)

Start by pouring the hot milk into a bowl. Add the chia seeds and stir. Let sit for 5 minutes, then stir briskly again to break up any lumps. Stir again after another 5 minutes, cover, and let soak for several hours or overnight. This allows the breakdown of any antinutrients (see note below), and makes the soaked seeds a lot more digestible and nutritious.

While your seeds are soaking, you can make the simple apple compôte. Put the apple in a small saucepan with a couple of tablespoons of water and the vanilla seeds. Place over medium heat with a tight-fitting lid. When it starts to bubble and steam, stir after a minute or two. It should take about 10 minutes to cook and break down. I like it still with some texture, not totally puréed. When it's softened, add the honey or date syrup to taste. At this point, reheat your chia pudding by placing it in a small saucepan with a tablespoon or 2 of water and warm through.

Scoop the pudding into two bowls and top with the apple compôte and a sprinkling of chopped pistachios or any other favorite nut. Toasted chopped almonds are delicious. If you have any borage flowers, they look beautiful sprinkled over. Serve while warm.

* Antinutrients are natural or synthetic compounds that interfere with the absorption of nutrients. They are found in the skins or coating of most seeds/nuts and grains. To neutralize the antinutrients, you can soak your seeds/nuts/grains for several hours or overnight. Times vary depending on what you are soaking.

BLACKBERRY & ROSE CHEESECAKE

with Flowers

This is a super fresh and decadent frozen cheesecake, a bit like an ice cream cake but healthy for you. It's easy to put together and really refreshing on a hot summer's evening for an outside dinner party. The crust is wonderfully chewy and nutty and the yogurt topping is everything it should be: fruity, fragrant, and creamy.

Serves 12

For the crust:
2 cups blanched almonds
⅓ cup sunflower seeds
12 fresh medjool dates, pitted
Zest of ½ lemon
2 tablespoons raw coconut oil
Hearty pinch of sea salt

For the filling:
1⅓ cups blackberries
⅔ cup blueberries
Juice of ½ lemon
½ cup raw honey
2½ cups Greek yogurt or
**   thick coconut yogurt**
1 teaspoon rose water

For the topping:
1¾ cups blackberries
⅔ cup blueberries

Flowers to decorate, preferably purple ones,
**   washed (must be unsprayed), (e.g. sweet peas,**
**   rose petals, lavender, cornflowers, violas)**

Preheat the oven to 350°F. Spread the almonds and sunflower seeds on a baking sheet and roast in the oven for about 6–8 minutes, or until they are starting to color a little and smell nutty. Remove from the oven and let cool a little.

Pour the nuts into a food processor and pulse just enough to chop them but do not let them become powdered. Add the dates, lemon zest, coconut oil, and a pinch of salt and process again until the mix comes together and you have a lovely looking sticky mixture.

Scrape the mixture into an 8 in nonstick, loose-bottomed cake pan and press it flat, but don't squish it. Place in the fridge to chill and set.

Purée the blackberries and blueberries in the food processor along with the lemon juice and honey. Scrape the mix into a large bowl and add the yogurt. Fold everything together until completely combined.

Spoon the topping over the chilled base and smooth it evenly using the back of a spoon. Put in the freezer and let it set for at least 3–4 hours. It needs to be frozen almost completely. The very middle is nice if it still has a bit of a wobble, but as it has no gelatin, it will not hold if it's not frozen. If you have frozen it overnight, move it to the fridge for half an hour before serving.

When you are ready to serve, simply bring the cheesecake out of the freezer (or fridge) and carefully unmold from the pan. Decorate with the extra berries and lots of petals.

A DECADENT CHOCOLATE MOUSSE

with Raspberry, Rose Compôte & Pistachios

You won't believe how simple it is to make this mousse, how delicious it tastes, and how amazingly good it is for you. Chocolate has a natural affinity for tart raspberries and the delicate floral notes of rose water. The pistachios add color and a pleasing crunch.

Serves 2–3

For the mousse:
⅓ **cup raw honey or maple syrup**
2 **ripe avocados**
1 **ripe banana**
Seeds from ½ **vanilla bean**
⅓ **cup raw cacao powder, plus extra for dusting (optional)**

For the compôte:
2½ **cups fresh raspberries**
Juice of ½ **lemon**
2 **tablespoons maple syrup or honey**
½ **teaspoon rose water**

To serve
¾ **cup pistachios, coarsely chopped**
Rose petals, washed (must be unsprayed), to decorate

To make the mousse, simply put all the ingredients into a powerful blender and process until you have a smooth mousse. If you want a lighter consistency, add a small splash of coconut water. Scrape into a serving bowl or individual bowls and put in the fridge to set, roughly 20 minutes.

Meanwhile, macerate your berries. Put the raspberries into a bowl, squeeze over the lemon juice, and pour in the syrup or honey and rose water. Mix well with a spoon, ever so lightly crushing the berries. Set aside for 10–15 minutes to macerate.

When the mousse is set and the berries are ready, simply spoon the berries over the mousse, top with chopped pistachios, and scatter a few petals over the top. A heavenly pudding—it's a feast for the eyes as well as the taste buds. Dust with more cacao powder, if you like.

COCONUT & APRICOT
BLISS BALLS

These wonderfully delicious little balls are perfect as a snack for packed lunches or an afternoon snack, or anytime for that matter. They last really well in the fridge, so once you have made a big batch they can be kept in the fridge for when you need them. They are light, moist, and can be coated with different things, which is great—you can coat some with nuts and some with seeds, and sometimes I like to coat some with freeze-dried berries—then you have some for all taste buds.

Makes approx. 40 balls

1½ cups sulphur-free dried apricots, plus 5 extra
1 medium mature coconut
Small handful of pistachios or cashews,
   coarsely chopped
1 generous tablespoon raw honey

To coat (use a few tablespoons of any of the following):
Sesame seeds
Shelled hemp seeds
Freeze-dried raspberries
Unsweetened, dried coconut flakes

First soak the dried apricots (except for the five extra) for 6–8 hours.

Make two holes in the coconut and drain the liquid through a fine strainer to catch any bits. Reserve the liquid for later use.

Break the shell open, scoop out the coconut flesh, and give it a quick rinse to wash off any pieces of shell. Cut the coconut flesh into pieces and put through a juicer.

Drain the soaked apricots and mix with the coconut pulp. Blend with an immersion blender or in a food processor (you could do this by hand if you mash and chop the soaked fruit really finely or use a large mortar and pestle). If the mix is too dry, spoon in a little reserved coconut water to bring it all together. Coarsely chop the five extra apricots and add it to the mixture along with the chopped nuts.

Use your hands to roll the mixture into small balls and then roll each one in your chosen coating. Place on a large tray or plate and transfer to the fridge to set.

These balls keep well in a cool place. Keep in the fridge until you're going to eat them.

RASPBERRY & ROSE
CUPCAKES

Sometimes life calls for something sweet, pretty, and delicious to mark an occasion. These are just the thing. Whether it's an afternoon snack or a picnic, they will impress. Sometimes I leave the frosting off and have them as breakfast muffins. Since they are full of nuts, fiber, and natural sweetening, they are a great way to kick-start the day. The cream topping doesn't last long, so they are best eaten soon after frosting them.

Makes 18
2¼ cups ground almonds
1 cup unsweetened, dried coconut flakes
1 large ripe banana, mashed
3 free-range eggs
¼ cup melted coconut oil, butter, or ghee
½ cup kefir, plain yogurt, or full-fat, well-blended coconut milk
10 medjool dates, pitted
1½ teaspoons baking powder (you can omit the baking powder if you don't mind a denser cupcake)
Seeds from ½ vanilla bean
1 teaspoon rose water
Pinch of sea salt
2 handfuls of fresh raspberries (red or white)

For the cream frosting:
Thick, Lovely Cashew Cream (see page 119), plus a handful of fresh raspberries
or
Light Coconut Cream with Vanilla (see page 118), plus a handful of fresh raspberries
or
Soft, Freshly Whipped Cream (see page 118), plus a handful of fresh raspberries

To serve
Rose petals, washed (must be unsprayed)
Small handful of pistachio nuts or almonds, coarsely chopped

Preheat the oven to 400°F. Line 18 cupcake molds with muffin cups.

Put all the ingredients for the cupcakes except the raspberries into a food processor and process until well-combined. Scrape the mixture into a bowl. (If you don't have a food processor, mash the bananas and dates to a soft mush, then add the rest of the ingredients except for the berries and beat with a wooden spoon until thoroughly combined.) Add the raspberries and gently stir through, then spoon the mixture into the prepared cups. Bake for 10–12 minutes, then remove from the oven and transfer to a wire rack to cool.

Meanwhile, prepare your chosen cream and push the raspberries through a strainer to remove the seeds. Fold the pulp and juices through the cream so that you have a lovely marbled effect.

Place dollops of cream on top of the cupcakes and decorate with fresh petals and chopped nuts.

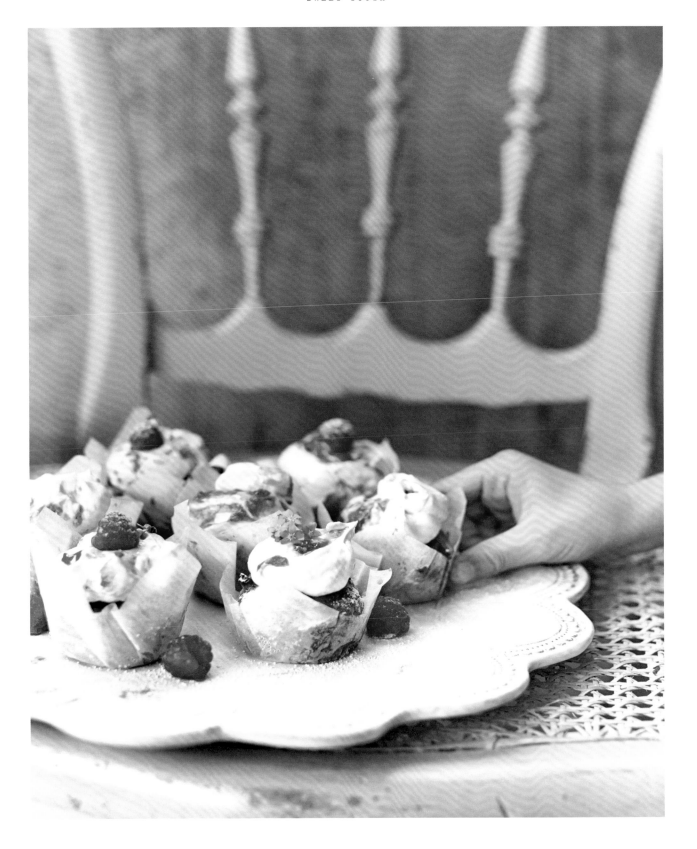

BAKED FIGS & STRAWBERRIES

with Honey, Vanilla & Toasted Almonds

Baked figs and strawberries are a match made in heaven, sweet and decadent. Eat as a dessert or for breakfast with some natural, unsweetened yogurt to balance the sweetness. This is best made in mid to late summer, when the figs are luscious and ripe and the end of the season's strawberries are full of flavor and bursting with sweetness. The almonds add crunch and texture. You can also serve this with Light Coconut Cream with Vanilla (see page 118) if you're not eating dairy.

Serves 6

1¼ lb perfectly ripe figs, stalks removed
7 tablespoons cold butter or raw cold coconut oil
1¾ cups in-season, smallish strawberries, hulled
½ cup raw or local honey (light honey is best)
Zest of 1 lemon and juice of ½ (can use an orange as a variation)
1 vanilla bean, seeds scraped out (or 1 teaspoon of vanilla essence)
1 cup sliced almonds

To serve
Yogurt or cream

Preheat the oven to 350°F.

Cut a cross in the top of each fig, then place them in a baking dish that will accommodate them all in a single layer, with a little extra room for the berries. Put a small pat of butter into the top of each fig and scatter with the strawberries. Drizzle the whole thing with the honey, squeeze over the lemon juice, dot with the vanilla seeds, and lastly sprinkle over the sliced almonds.

Bake in the oven until the figs are just collapsing, about 10–15 minutes. Take the dish out of the oven and sprinkle with the lemon zest. Serve hot or warm with your favorite yogurt or cream.

SPICED CHOCOLATE &
SWEET POTATO BROWNIES

These gluten-free brownies can be eaten just as they are for a delicious snack, or they can be plated for a special dessert and served with a spoonful of crème fraîche, a dusting of raw cacao powder, and perhaps a few fresh raspberries.

Makes 16
3 medium sweet potatoes
12 fresh medjool dates, pitted
¾ cup ground almonds
⅔ cup buckwheat flour
3 tablespoons raw cacao nibs
¼ cup raw cacao powder, plus extra to serve
3 tablespoons honey
Zest of 1 orange
½ teaspoon ground cinnamon

Preheat the oven to 350°F and line a 9 × 13 in brownie pan or baking dish.

Peel your sweet potatoes, put them into a steamer, and steam for about 18–20 minutes or until completely soft. Remove them from the steamer and transfer to a food processor along with the pitted dates and blend.

Mix the remaining ingredients in a large bowl, then add the sweet potato and date mixture to the bowl and fold everything together.

Spoon the mixture into the lined pan and cook for about 20 minutes. Remove from the oven and let cool a little before dusting with raw cacao powder, cutting, and serving.

BERRY & ROSE COCONUT ICE CREAM

Blackcurrants have quite an intense flavor, so this one is more for the adults (unless your child likes slightly sour, tart flavors... some do!) The rose goes beautifully with the blackcurrants. I tend to like my currants quite tart but if you like them sweeter, just add a bit more honey. These little black berries have gone a bit out of fashion but I think they are marvelous things, full of vitamin C and such a rich, deep purple color, which contrasts so beautifully with pink rose petals and the emerald green of the pistachio.

Serves 3–4
⅔ cup blackberries, frozen
⅔ cup blueberries, frozen
¾ cup full-fat coconut milk
2 tablespoons raw honey
1 teaspoon rose water

To serve
Small dark pink rose petals, washed
  (must be unsprayed)
Handful of pistachios, finely chopped

Place all the ingredients into a food processor and process until you have a soft ice cream. Scoop into bowls, top with rose petals and chopped pistachios, and serve immediately.

BANANA & RAW CACAO ICE CREAM

with Pomegranates & Cacao Nibs

This is a really nourishing and decadent treat. The cacao nibs and pomegranate seeds add a lovely contrasting crunch to its super creamy texture. The raw cacao powder and nibs are quite bitter, which is how I love my chocolate.

Serves 2–4
4 ripe bananas, sliced into thin rounds
2 tablespoons raw cacao powder
½ cup unsweetened almond milk
2 tablespoons maple syrup

To serve
Seeds from 1 pomegranate
2 tablespoons raw cacao nibs

First put your banana slices in a large plastic bag in the freezer. Lay the bag flat so that the banana slices don't freeze in one big clump; I usually leave mine in the freezer overnight, but they will only take a few hours.

When the slices are thoroughly frozen, put them into a food processor or high-speed blender with the cacao powder, almond milk, and syrup and process for 1–2 minutes, scraping down the sides as necessary. The bananas will thaw a little, melting beautifully into the other components to make that delicious velvety smooth ice cream texture.

Once you have the right consistency, scrape the ice cream into several dessert bowls, sprinkle with pomegranate seeds and raw cacao nibs, and serve at once.

FROZEN YOGURT
& BLACKBERRY SWIRL POPS

These make for an impressive treat. They are great to make with the kids, perfect for parties or summer barbecues, or just after-school snacks. They are super healthy but super yummy, and kids love them (so do I).

Makes 8
1½ **cups blackberries**
⅓ **cup honey, plus an extra 1½ tablespoons**
2 **cups plain yogurt**

8 **small disposable plastic cups**
8 **wooden sticks**

Combine the blackberries and the honey in a small saucepan over low heat. Simmer so that the berries cook down and start to become syrupy.

Remove the pan from the heat and process the berries with an immersion blender, then pass through a strainer into a clean bowl. Set aside to cool.

Mix the yogurt and the 1½ tablespoons of honey in a separate large bowl. Gently fold half the cooled berry mix into the yogurt to create a swirl.

Spoon the mix equally into the plastic cups, pouring a little extra of the purée into the middle of each one. Place the cups on a shallow pan, cover with foil, then stick your wooden sticks through the foil into the center of each cup. The foil will help keep the sticks in place while the pops are freezing. Place the pan in the freezer and freeze for 3–4 hours or until ready to serve. Run the bottom of each cup under hot water to loosen the pop.

A SUMMERY POMEGRANATE
& STRAWBERRY CAKE

*Here's a sugar-free cake for celebratory occasions. It's light, fruity, creamy, and perfect for
a summery afternoon when the strawberries are sweet and fragrant.*

Serves 8–10

2 sticks + 5 tablespoons unsalted butter, softened
2½ cups white spelt flour, sifted
4 medium free-range eggs
3 level teaspoons baking powder
2 teaspoons rose water
1 cup maple syrup
Grated zest of 1 lemon
2–3 tablespoons kefir or milk to loosen the mix

For the filling:
1¾ cups heavy cream
2 tablespoons maple syrup
1 teaspoon rose water
¼ cup Greek-style plain yogurt or kefir
**6 tablespoons rose petal jam or sugar-free
  strawberry jam**
1 pomegranate, halved and seeds removed
Squeeze of lemon juice
1¾ cups strawberries

Preheat the oven to 350°F. Grease and flour 3 × 8 in loose-bottomed cake pans.

In a large mixing bowl, cream the butter until pale and fluffy with a hand-held mixer. Add 2–3 tablespoons of the flour and beat in the eggs, one at a time, and beat until you have a light, fluffy mixture (if it looks like it's curdling, add another tablespoon of flour). Using a large metal spoon, gently fold in the remaining flour and baking powder until just combined; don't overmix. Add the rose water, maple syrup, and lemon zest and fold in gently. Add a dash of kefir or milk to loosen if too stiff.

Divide the mixture between the pans, level the top with a palette knife, and bake in the oven for 20 minutes or until the center springs back to the touch. Remove from the oven and cool in the pans for 5–10 minutes before turning onto a wire rack to cool completely.

Meanwhile, make the filling. Whip the cream until it forms soft peaks, then gently stir through the maple syrup and rose water. Fold in the yogurt or kefir, then carefully dot spoonfuls of jam into the cream bowl and stir gently to create a lovely marble effect.

Place one cake layer on a serving plate, gently spoon the cream mixture over the top, and sprinkle with pomegranate seeds. Top with the second cake layer, decorate with marbled cream and pomegranate seeds, then repeat a third time with the remaining layer.

Lastly, top the cake with your strawberries and sprinkle with any remaining pomegranate seeds. You can also crush a few pomegranate seeds and flick the juice over the cake—this gives a lovely effect.

TOOLBOX

This is my go-to selection of basics: mayos, dressings, dips, sauces, and more. You won't believe how easy it is to make these basic things, and nothing you buy in the supermarket will compare. I have yet to find a comparable pesto sauce from a jar; personally, I don't think it exists. However, if you prepare your own, you can make sure the best and freshest ingredients go into the mix, and end up with something truly health-giving and totally delicious. Mayonnaise has had a bit of a bad reputation, and when I think of jarred mayo, I can understand why; I urge you to try making your own. It's so incredibly good for you, full of healthy fats and proteins. It lasts for a good few days in the fridge and really isn't as tricky as everyone tells you. If you find it splitting, simply add a tablespoon of warm water and keep going; it should spring back, no problem.

You can play around with different olive oils for varying degrees of greenness and fruitiness. There are lots of delicious dressings in this chapter that are perfect for enhancing any type of salad you want to serve.

GREMOLATA

I love this stuff: it totally rocks! Anything with gremolata will pop and sing. One small sprinkle elevates the plain to totally genius. I add it to pretty much everything: soups, salads, open sandwiches, and roasted vegetables—particularly carrots, parsnips, squash, and sweet potatoes. You can also use it on meat before or after roasting fish and chicken. I love it every which way. What's more, it's a great way of using up any parsley that would ordinarily get left in the vegetable drawer of your fridge and inevitably be thrown away, and how many times have we all done that?

Serves enough to sprinkle on a recipe for 4
**Bunch of parsley, leaves picked
  and finely chopped**
**1 big fat garlic clove or 2 small ones,
  finely chopped**
Zest of 2 lemons

Simply place all the components into a bowl and toss. That's it, so simple. It keeps well in the fridge for a couple of days, but make sure it's sealed with plastic wrap or in an airtight jar.

Variation
My mother grows the most delicious mustard greens. I used to wander through her garden and pick all the baby salad leaves, and mustard greens were one of my favorites, deliciously mustardy and peppery. Use them in place of the parsley in the gremolata recipe for a different note.

TARRAGON GREMOLATA

3 tablespoons finely chopped tarragon leaves
Zest of 1 lemon
½ garlic clove, finely chopped

Combine all the ingredients in a small bowl. It will last for only about a day.

HUMMUS

Hummus is a great thing; kids love it, adults love it. I don't know anyone who doesn't. There are some really good ones you can buy, but I much prefer the taste of homemade hummus, and that way I know it contains the best quality oils, so no bad fats. Bad fats are one of the worst thing for anyone to eat, especially children. However, homemade hummus gives you the best of everything, and it tastes much better.

Serves 6

1 × 14 oz can chickpeas (preferably from a glass jar), drained

¼ cup (or more) lemon juice

4 garlic cloves, finely grated

2 teaspoons cumin

Salt to taste

¾ cup tahini

½ cup water

¼ cup extra virgin olive oil, plus a little extra for drizzling

2 teaspoons smoked paprika

2 tablespoons finely chopped curly parsley

Place everything except the paprika and parsley into a blender and process until smooth—or put everything in a bowl and use an immersion blender, which saves you from cleaning up the blender.

Once the mixture is lovely and creamy, spoon it into a bowl then, using the back of the spoon, carefully smooth it out, creating a pretty swirl on the top. Sprinkle with the paprika and parsley, then drizzle a little oil on top.

ROASTED RED PEPPER HUMMUS WITH CHIPOTLE

Prepare the hummus (as left), but omit the water and add the flesh of 2 roasted red bell peppers, skins and seeds removed. Replace the cumin and paprika and parsley with 1½ teaspoons of chipotle powder.

Finish as left but sprinkle with a little extra chipotle powder.

ROASTED SQUASH & ROSEMARY HUMMUS

Prepare the hummus (as left) but omit the water and add 1 cup of roasted butternut squash.

Finish as left but sprinkle with a few rosemary leaves instead of the paprika and parsley.

KALE CRISPS

Kale crisps are perfectly delicious and yet so easy to make. The key is not to have any water on the leaves; if there is moisture they will just wilt in the oven, so I tend to wash the leaves the night before and then leave them on the counter on a clean kitchen towel to dry. You will be surprised how easy these are if you haven't made them before, and a lot cheaper than buying them in a store.

Makes a generous bowlful
1 bunch of kale, 8–10 big leaves
1 tablespoon olive oil
¼ teaspoon sea salt

Optional flavorings:
Warming mix
¼ teaspoon turmeric
¼ teaspoon ground cumin
¼ teaspoon ground coriander

Spicy mix
¼ teaspoon chipotle powder
¼ teaspoon oregano

Preheat the oven to 275°F and line a baking sheet with parchment paper.

Wash the kale leaves and dry them VERY well. Using a paring knife, scissors, or simply your hands, strip or cut out and discard the center stem.

Cut the leaves into 2 in pieces. Put them in a bowl, drizzle with olive oil, and sprinkle with the salt. Massage the oil and salt into the leaves until they are well coated with a thin layer of oil. At this point, you can either keep them plain or sprinkle on one of the spice mixes. Spread the kale out on the baking sheet and transfer to the oven for 8–12 minutes or until just crisp.

Some of the leaves may crisp faster than others, so take out any that are done, then continue cooking the rest until they are all crisp. They can be eaten right away or stored for several days in an airtight container.

KIMCHI

*Kimchi, like sauerkraut, is fermented and very good for you, full of enzymes and
probiotics that boost immunity and aid digestion. Try to find Korean red pepper flakes for
their slightly sweet, smoky flavor, but otherwise use any red pepper flakes you can find.*

Makes 1 large 2.5 liter jar

**1 large Chinese cabbage (also known as Napa
cabbage), quartered lengthwise, inner cores
removed**

2½ tablespoons sea salt

**Several quarts spring water, or mineral water
(not tap water—the chlorine will stop the
fermentation process)**

1 daikon, peeled and cut into matchsticks

4 scallions, trimmed and cut into 2 in pieces

For the paste

**1 tablespoon grated garlic
(about 5 or 6 medium cloves)**

1 teaspoon grated fresh ginger

1 teaspoon unrefined sugar

¼ cup fish sauce (a good quality one)

1–5 tablespoons Korean red pepper flakes

Equipment

**A large 2.5 liter glass jar, sterilized
(boil for 10 minutes on the rack of a
boiling-water canner)**

Cut each cabbage quarter across into 1¼ in strips
and put in a large bowl. Gently massage the salt into
the cabbage until it starts to soften a little—1 or 2
minutes. Add water to cover the cabbage. Put a plate
on top to weigh it down. Set aside for 1–2 hours. Pour
off the brine into a separate bowl and reserve. Rinse
the cabbage under cold water, then let it sit for about
10 minutes in a colander to dry off—pat dry with paper
towels to remove excess water. Set aside.

For the paste, combine the garlic, ginger, sugar, and
fish sauce in small bowl. Mix in the Korean red pepper
flakes, using 1 tablespoon for mild or 5 (or more!) for a
fiery taste.

Next take the large bowl used to salt your cabbage,
make sure it is clean, and put in all the vegetables
and the paste. Mix with your hands, massaging the
seasoning into the vegetables really well. (Use gloves to
protect your hands from pepper flakes, stains or odors.)

Pack the kimchi into a jar, pressing it down well. Pour
in enough of the reserved brine to cover the vegetables
completely—it needs to be under the brine. Allow 1½ in
headspace at the top of the jar. Seal and let it stand at
room temperature for 3–5 days, or longer if you're feeling
brave! You will see bubbles inside and brine may seep
out at the top, so put it in a bowl to catch any overflow.
Once a day, press down the vegetables to keep them
submerged; this releases the gases during fermentation.
Taste it daily to check for desired sourness and ripeness.

When the kimchi is to your liking, store the jar in the
fridge. You can eat it right away, but it's better if you
leave it for a couple of weeks.

MAYONNAISE

Mayo got a bad name after the awful store-bought varieties were slathered over even more awful soggy sandwiches. And most of those you buy are terrible for one's health (full of bad fats), in complete contrast to the delicious homemade version (full of good fats). Homemade mayo is actually incredibly good for you, as long as you use the right ingredients: cold-pressed oils and organic free-range eggs—those are good fats with omegas—and in the right ratio. There are SO many delicious ways to use mayo: salads, roast chicken, fish, roasted veggies, oven-roasted fries, fish cakes, crab, you name it…

Makes 1½ cups
2 organic free-range egg yolks
1 teaspoon Dijon mustard
½ tablespoon apple cider vinegar
  or a squeeze of lemon
⅔ cup extra virgin olive oil
⅔ cup cold-pressed sunflower or canola oil
Sea salt and freshly ground pepper

I usually make my mayo by hand, which is easier than you think and saves you from washing lots of equipment.

Position a large bowl on a damp cloth on your work surface to hold it in place. Put the egg yolks in the bowl, add the mustard or lemon juice and vinegar, and whisk with a balloon whisk to combine.

Combine the two oils in a separate bowl. Pour a very small amount of the oil, only a drop or two, to the yolks and whisk until it's thoroughly combined, then add a tiny bit more oil and whisk again. Keep going in this fashion until quite a bit of oil is incorporated, which should only take about 3–4 minutes, then start adding more oil at a time. Once I have incorporated the first few drops of oil I add it in a steady trickle with one hand and whisk with the other, stopping every so often to give it a really good whisk before starting the steady trickle again. Once the desired consistency is reached, stop adding the oil (you may not need it all, depending on how you like your mayo). If the mayo starts to split (separate) or you want to thin it a little, add a small amount of warm water.

Now taste it and season as you like it. You can adjust the flavor by adding a little more of the vinegar (or lemon juice) or mustard. It keeps for up to a week in the fridge.

APPLE CIDER VINEGAR

& Raw Honey

This is really good, and my go-to dressing for just about any kind of salad or side dish. It keeps very well for a long time.

1 garlic clove, finely grated
1 heaping teaspoon Dijon mustard
¼ cup apple cider vinegar
2 tablespoons lemon juice
1–2 tablespoons raw honey
  (start with one then add
  more if you like)
⅓ cup extra virgin olive oil
Sea salt and freshly ground
  pepper to taste

Put everything in a jar with a tight-fitting lid or a bowl and either shake or whisk until completely emulsified.

SIMPLEST EVER OLIVE OIL

& Lemon Juice Dressing

This one is for when you just need a little something extra on your vegetables, but not a full-blown dressing. It's very good and incredibly alkalizing.

¼ cup extra virgin olive oil
3 tablespoons lemon juice
Sea salt and freshly ground
  pepper to taste

Simply whisk the oil and lemon in a bowl, season to taste, and use immediately.

JAPANESE DRESSING

This one is something a bit different: try it on steamed vegetables or a carrot and beet salad or Roast Pumpkin, Golden Beet & Squash Salad (see page 59).

½ cup red onion, finely chopped
3 tablespoons soy sauce
2 tablespoons rice wine vinegar
½ teaspoon raw honey or maple
  syrup
¼ teaspoon English mustard
  powder
1 tablespoon grapeseed oil
1 tablespoon sesame oil
Sea salt and freshly ground
  pepper to taste

Put everything in a jar with a tight-fitting lid, shake really well until completely emulsified, then add 2 tablespoons of water. Taste and season accordingly.

These dressings all make enough for one big salad.

BLACK OLIVE

& Olive Oil Dressing

This is a niçoise dressing for Salade Niçoise, but since it's quite punchy, it goes really well with other bold salads, potatoes, fish, and plenty of other delicious things.

⅓ **cup black olives, pitted**
5 **good-quality marinated anchovy fillets**
1 **garlic clove**
Juice of ½ **lemon**
¼ **cup olive oil**
1 **tablespoon apple cider vinegar**

Put the olives, anchovies, and garlic into a large mortar and mash with a pestle to make a rough paste. Scrape the mix into a bowl, stir in the lemon juice, olive oil, and vinegar, and set aside for 10–30 minutes before using so that the flavors can really develop.

ORANGE BLOSSOM

& Maple Syrup Dressing

This dressing is truly amazing on any kind of salad with fruit in it. It really comes alive with the floral notes from the orange blossom water. Be sure to use original Lebanese brands like Cortas, which you can find online. Supermarket brands are much more intense so, if using, start by adding ½ teaspoon at a time.

1 **tablespoon orange blossom water**
2 **tablespoons apple cider vinegar**
1 **tablespoon maple syrup**
3 **tablespoons olive oil**
Juice of ½ **lemon**
½ **garlic clove, finely grated**
Sea salt and freshly ground pepper to taste

Combine all the ingredients and whisk in a bowl or shake in a jar with a tight-fitting lid until completely emulsified. Let stand for 10 minutes or more before using to allow the flavors to come together.

FRESH ORANGE DRESSING

Another great salad dressing for fruity salads and bitter leaf salads.

Zest and juice of 2 oranges
1 **tablespoon apple cider vinegar**
1 **teaspoon raw honey**
Pinch of sea salt and a few twists of freshly ground black pepper
½ **cup extra virgin olive oil**

Put the orange zest and juice in a mixing bowl and stir in the vinegar, honey, salt, and pepper. Slowly pour in the oil, a little at a time, whisking continuously to bring it together.

YOGURT SAUCE

with herb spices

This little gem is as amazing with grilled meats and roast chicken as it is with roasted vegetables and a salad. It will make any plate sing.

Enough for 4 as an accompaniment
1¾ **cups Greek or plain yogurt**
2 **large garlic cloves, crushed or finely grated**
1 **green chile, seeded and finely chopped**
6–8 **tablespoons finely chopped dill, stalks removed**
Sea salt and freshly ground black pepper to taste

Simply put all the ingredients in a bowl and combine. Allow to amalgamate for 15 minutes before using to allow all the flavors to really mingle. Taste before serving as often the seasoning will need to be adjusted.

VEGETABLE STOCK

Making your own vegetable stock is really worth the effort. If you're making soups, casseroles, or risottos, it's the magic ingredient. It's super easy, makes a great vegetable broth, and is very restorative and healing.

Makes a big bowlful
4 **garlic cloves**
2 **onions, quartered**
3 **carrots, cut into chunks**
2 **stalks of celery, each cut into 4 pieces**
1 **large leek, cut into chunks**
Handful of flat-leaf parsley
4 **sprigs of thyme**
2 **sprigs of tarragon**
2 **bay leaves**
1½ **teaspoons salt**
1 **teaspoon black peppercorns**

Place everything into a big pot, cover with 3½–4 quarts of water, bring to a boil, then reduce the heat and simmer for an hour. Let the stock cool and pour through a strainer, discard all the solids, and store the broth in jars in the fridge or freezer.

ROASTED RED PEPPER & ROSEMARY SPREAD

This is so easy to make and totally grain-free. I first came across the idea in The Green Kitchen *by David Frenkiel and Luise Vindahl, and this is my version. I love to keep a jar of it in my fridge at all times—it's perfect with roasted or raw vegetables, a grilled piece of fish, or as a spread on rye toast with avocado and salad. The seeds add lots of good oils, particularly the pumpkin seeds, which have lots of zinc that helps to balance the hormones and clear the skin.*

Makes 1 × 18 oz jar
3 red bell peppers, seeded and halved
Olive oil
2 sprigs of rosemary, leaves picked
⅓ cup sunflower seeds
⅓ cup pumpkin seeds
Pinch of smoked paprika
Juice of ½ lemon
A hearty pinch of sea salt and freshly
**   ground black pepper**

Preheat your oven to 400°F.

Place the prepared peppers onto a flat roasting pan and drizzle with olive oil. Sprinkle with the rosemary and toss. Roast for about 40 minutes or until slightly charred at the edges and the skin is easy to peel off. Set aside to cool.

Next, lightly toast the seeds in a dry frying pan until they start to release their delicious nutty aroma and begin to pop. Transfer them to a bowl.

When the peppers are cool enough to handle, peel off the skins. Place them into a bowl along with the rest of the ingredients and process until smooth. Taste and adjust the seasoning if necessary. Scrape your mix into a sterilized glass jar and keep in the fridge for up to 2 weeks, if it lasts that long!! Mine never does.

DUKKAH

This Egyptian spice blend is glorious sprinkled onto an omelet or scrambled eggs, or on avocado on toast. It goes well on roast chicken, or with fish. Serve a small bowlful alongside one with good quality olive oil and a pile of fresh, hot whole-grain pita bread. It keeps for ages on the shelf in an airtight jar, but it's so good it won't be around for long.

Makes 1 medium jarful
1 cup hazelnuts
6 tablespoons coriander seeds
6 teaspoons sesame seeds
4 tablespoons cumin seeds
2 tablespoons black peppercorns
2 teaspoons fennel seeds
2 teaspoons dried mint leaves
2 teaspoons flaky sea salt

Heat a heavy-bottomed pan over high heat, add the hazelnuts, and dry roast until slightly browned and fragrant, being careful not to let them burn, which they can do easily. Remove from the heat and cool completely.

Repeat the procedure with each of the seeds and peppercorns, making sure you cool each completely.

Place the nuts, seeds, mint, and salt into a mortar or small spice blender and pound or pulse until the mix is a coarse consistency. Do NOT allow the mix to become a paste; you want a crumbly spice mix. Delicious.

MY MOM'S PLUM SAUCE

This is the sauce I grew up on. I LOVE it!! If I had to choose five favorite tastes from my childhood, this would be one of them. We had it on everything from fish and chips to Shepherd's Pie, or with our delicious homemade sausages. My mom always had the shelves stocked with this sauce. It's like a plum version of a tomato sauce, rather than the thick sweet Chinese plum sauce. Use it as you would ketchup. Half the recipe is good for the first time until you're addicted, like me!

Makes enough to last you 6 months
7½ lbs dark red tart plums, halved and pitted
6⅔ cups unrefined organic golden granulated sugar
2 teaspoons sea salt
1 teaspoon allspice berries
1 teaspoon whole cloves
1 cup grated fresh ginger
2 quarts apple cider vinegar

Place everything into a large, heavy-bottomed pot, bring to a boil, and simmer for 2 hours. Set aside to cool completely. When it's cooled to room temperature, pour into sterilized bottles with sealing lids or tops. This sauce will keep well for months if sealed properly.

PESTO

a few ways

Pesto is great as a dip, as sauce for roasted vegetables, as a dressing or on sandwiches, even on rye toast with a delicious soft cheese. It's full of good fats to feed the brain and herbs that aid digestion and give many micronutrients that feed the body on a deep level.

CLASSIC PESTO

Makes enough for 3–4
½ garlic clove, chopped
3 handfuls of basil leaves, chopped
1 handful of pinenuts, lightly toasted
1 hearty handful of Parmesan (or a mature Pecorino), finely grated
⅔ cup extra virgin olive oil
Small squeeze of lemon juice
Sea salt and freshly ground black pepper

Add the garlic, basil, pine nuts, Parmesan, and olive oil to a food processor and process it to a rough sauce; I don't like it too smooth. You can add a little extra oil if you like it more runny. Add a squeeze of lemon, just a small one, and season to taste.

WALNUT PESTO WITH BASIL OR KALE

Makes enough for 3–4
1¾ cups walnut halves or pieces
1 garlic clove
Handful of basil (or kale)
1 cup Parmesan, freshly grated
½ cup extra virgin olive oil
Sea salt and freshly ground black pepper

Place everything into a blender and process until you have a coarse sauce. Adjust the balance with a little extra cheese or oil. Season to taste.

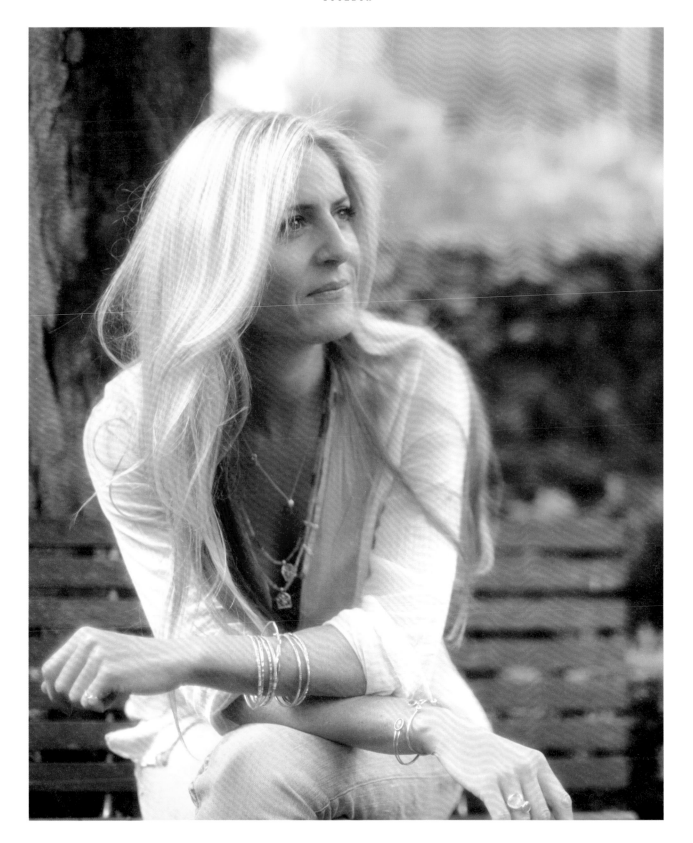

SOFT, FRESHLY WHIPPED CREAM

This is perfect for topping fruit pies and or other desserts, fruit salad with a sprinkle of my rose water Granola (see page 40), or even as a topping for my Coconut and Banana Pancakes (see page 33) with a sugar-free jam. You can use this cream in so many ways.

2 cups fresh cream
3 tablespoons plain yogurt
   or kefir
2 tablespoons raw honey or raw
   date syrup (see page 119)

Whip the cream to ribbon consistency, then gently fold in the yogurt or kefir and honey or syrup with a spatula. If you like your cream a little stiffer, just beat a little more until you achieve the desired thickness, but don't overwhip.

RICH MASCARPONE CREAM

This is good with baked fruits hot from the oven, because it will melt into the hot fruit and create a lovely melty sauce—total heaven! It's also good on cakes as a frosting.

2 cups mascarpone or sour cream
3 free-range egg yolks
⅓ cup maple syrup, raw honey, or
   raw date syrup (see page 119)

Beat the mascarpone lightly in a bowl. Beat the egg yolks in a separate bowl and slowly add the maple syrup, honey, or date syrup. Fold in the mascarpone. Chill in the fridge.

LIGHT COCONUT CREAM

with Vanilla

Use this as you would the softly whipped cow's cream. It's great for people who are avoiding dairy, it's vegan friendly, and it tastes totally indulgent! I love eating this with my Som Tum Pollamai fruit salad (see page 47).

1 × 14 oz can full-fat coconut milk
1 teaspoon raw honey or raw date
   syrup (see page 119), or to taste
Seeds from ¼ vanilla bean

Place the can of coconut milk upside down in the fridge for several hours or overnight. Turn the can the right-side up, open, and pour off the thin coconut water into a bowl or small jar and set aside for another use.

Spoon out the thick cream in the bottom of the can into a medium bowl, add the honey or date syrup and vanilla seeds, then whip with a whisk or beat with a hand-held mixer for about 3–5 minutes until light and fluffy like whipped cream. If it's too thick, you can add 1–2 teaspoons of the reserved coconut water to make it lighter and smoother. Taste and add more honey or date syrup, if you like.

THICK, LOVELY CASHEW CREAM

This cream is really velvety and nutty and creamy—totally luscious. It's a great non-dairy alternative but even if you are having dairy I still choose this sometimes; it's a treat unto itself. It's beautiful with baked fruits and on top of cakes.

1¼ **cups cashew nuts, soaked for at least 4 hours or overnight**
1–2 **tablespoons raw honey or date syrup (see right), or to taste**
Seeds from ¼ vanilla bean
Pinch of sea salt
½ **cup water**

Put the cashew nuts, 1 tablespoon of the honey or date syrup, the vanilla seeds, and salt into a high-speed blender. Add two-thirds of the water and pulse, scraping down the sides if necessary, until it's lovely and velvety and smooth. If it's too thick, add more water to thin it out to the desired consistency. Taste and add more honey or date syrup, if you like.

Variation
For a fruit version of any of these creams, use a fork to mash a few perfectly ripe in-season berries—raspberries, blackberries, or blueberries all work well, strawberries less so; (they're too watery)—then marble them through the cream before serving. If you don't like the seeds, mash the fruit with a fork, then push the mix through a strainer, discard the seeds, and marble the pulp and liquid through the cream.

RAW DATE SYRUP

Medjool dates have a deep, sweet flavor that makes them a perfect alternative to processed sugar when you need a natural sweetener.

10 **medjool dates, pitted (or 20 normal dates, pitted)**
1¾ **cups lukewarm water**
1 **teaspoon fresh lemon juice**

Start by soaking the dates in the water overnight, covered. Then place them in a blender along with the soaking water and lemon juice. Process until completely smooth. Transfer to a jar with a lid and store in the fridge; it keeps for up to 3 weeks.

NUT MILK

This is a great alternative to dairy milk. It's easy to make and so delicious.

1 **cup almonds**
Up to 2 cups fresh water (filtered or spring water is best)

Start by soaking the nuts in a bowl overnight. The water should cover the nuts by at least an inch. The next day, drain the nuts and place them in a blender. Process them for 2 minutes.

Take a piece of cheesecloth or a nut milk bag and place it over a bowl. Pour in the nut milk mixture and then, with clean hands, squeeze the liquid through the cloth into the bowl, extracting as much milk as possible. You should have about 2 cups of milk. You now have ground almonds left in the cloth, which you can use for baking.

Pour your nut milk into a jar with a lid and store in the fridge to keep it cool until you are ready to use it. It will last in the fridge for a couple of days, but you will need to give it a good shake before using.

SUPER WOMAN

Sadie

From my earliest memories, diet and exercise have been very important to me. Taking care of my body has been a very natural process that has come easily, so in some ways I have been lucky. I was a natural vegetarian from the start; as a child I chose not to eat meat because I intensely disliked the taste of both meat and fish. My childhood was spent exercising, dancing, and doing gymnastics, always pushing myself to the limit. All of this physical activity gave me a great start and a solid foundation for living healthily.

I've always strived to do my best, to challenge myself, and to try my utmost to be positive and content. Of course, as I have found out, getting a certain amount of balance in life isn't always easy and it is quite possible to lose your way and become disillusioned and unmotivated. Life doesn't always bring contentment, happiness, and peace of mind. For every one of us it's a journey: we can be up or down, we can be happy or sad, positive or negative. So many people suffer from anxiety, depression, and/or feelings of worthlessness at some point in life and I too have experienced all of these, which led me to explore many avenues to find some contentment.

I wanted to use my part of the book to outline how I conquered my demons. My aim is to share what I have learned from my experience in an approachable and unintimidating way…

I wanted to use my part of the book to outline how I conquered my demons. My aim is to share what I have learned from my experience in an approachable and unintimidating way, giving you the same insights I have gained from those who have taught and helped me over the years.

To live in the moment is vital. I used to spend so much of my life rushing around, never present, never listening, always on the phone or distracted. Listening is a very important skill and something I have always had to work on. Even normal human functions were a strain—eating, sleeping, and just living were all tasks that I found very difficult. How, I wondered, could I change? I ate right, I exercised and, yet, it still felt like there was something wrong with me. I saw healers, homeopaths, acupuncturists, gurus, and meditation experts. The number of specialists I visited was endless—a full-time job really! But each time I saw someone I took a little bit of their thinking away with me and eventually I put together my own little plan for mind, body, and soul that I now try to practice every day. It's a plan that fits into my normal routine because I am a working mom with a lot going on, not someone living on a mountain or taking time out on a yoga retreat. Of course, I am far from perfect and sometimes my plan falls apart into a million pieces. But each time this happens it is becoming easier to pick myself up, dust myself off, and start again.

When you experience peace of mind and contentment, it is the most wonderful feeling in the world, as if warm honey is running through your veins. There is a certain detachment, a sitting back and letting go. You feel alert, yet slightly fuzzy, like on one of those perfect summer days when you feel totally blissed out and loved. You can sit and listen to people and take it all in, without your mind churning through pointless thoughts.

The plan I have developed uses a combination of yoga, meditation, mindfulness, and good eating. It is a daily practice of positivity, assertiveness, and surrender that nurtures the mind, body, and soul and it begins with the way you breathe.

Love,
Sadie x

BREATH

Breath is everything! It gives us energy, life, and, if we are breathing properly, contentment and calmness. We can go for some time without water, food, and sleep, but breath is essential. How we breathe can rapidly rejuvenate us and connect us to our life-force. In yoga practice, "breath" is called "pranayama," "prana" meaning life force and "yama" extension. So the translation of pranayama is "extension of life-force." It can help engage our body and mind in times of need.

As a young child I suffered from a condition called bronchiectasis, which meant I had breathing difficulties. I was subjected to panic attacks and anxiety because I was not truly connected to my breath. Once I started to learn how important it was to breathe properly, I became calmer and more in control and at peace with myself. Over the years, I have learned many breathing techniques from lots of people, from voice coaches, singing teachers, and finally from some of the best yoga teachers I could find, which was when I really began to understand breath and the power of it. When you control the inhalation and exhalation of breath, it purifies and cleans your body. Immediately breathing can calm your mind and at the same time give you energy.

When I wake up in the morning, I slowly open my eyes. I try to focus on the moment, not on the hectic day I may have ahead of me. I start by engaging with pranayama and a light meditation along with some of my favorite mantras, saying something such as "I am content in the now" or "I love and support myself." This means I start my day in a serene, calm, and connected way and, hopefully, my whole day will be focused and enjoyable. I really notice a difference; I have clarity of thought and I am calm. If I don't do this it can be a whole other story, which sees me rushing around like a headless chicken worrying about the kids and my busy schedule.

So, in a very simple way, I will explain how I use my breath in some exercises.

TYPES *of* BREATH

Ujjayi (u-jai-yee)

Ujjayi, meaning hissing, is one of my favorite types of breath. It is also called the sounding breath due to the huffing sound you make as you exhale. When I breathe in this way, it makes me feel energized, focused, and improves my concentration in the physical practice. Becoming absorbed in Ujjayi allows you to remain in a yoga pose for longer periods of time. It also enhances more of a flow to the practice. Ujjayi breathing is also beneficial for respiratory conditions such as asthma and bronchitis.

Sit up straight, close your eyes, and breath naturally.

When you are ready to begin, take a deep breath in through your nose. Let the breath flow through your body. As you exhale, constrict your throat slightly so that there is a tension there, and then release the breath from the tension in your throat to create a *haaa* sound. Imagine you are cleaning a pair of glasses and huff on the lense, as it is a similar action and sound.

Inhale again and, as you did before, let the tension in your throat create the same *haaa* sound as you exhale. Once you have got the hang of this, close your mouth and breathe through your nostrils. You should now start to sound like Darth Vader!

Once you have mastered this on the exhale, use the tension in your throat to create the same breath and sound on the inhale too. (You truly will sound like Darth Vader now!)

Breath of Fire

Breath of Fire is a breathing technique that is used to boost your energy as it oxygenates and detoxifies the blood. It also aids brain function and concentration. It is great for calming the nervous system and for giving a sense of well-being, although some recommend not to practice it if you are pregnant or menstruating. The best time to perform breath of fire is in the morning, or a few hours after eating when your food has digested.

To begin, take some normal deep breaths, then start to inhale and exhale rapidly through your nose, keeping the length of the inhale and exhale equal. You will notice your stomach contract with some force.

Another way to start is by sticking your tongue out and panting like a dog. Then close your mouth and continue breath and rhythm, rapidly inhaling and exhaling through your nose. This sets up a good rhythm to stick with. Use your abdomen to inhale and exhale, pulling it in tightly and then pumping out the air just like using a set of bellows.

For best results, try to practice Breath of Fire for 1–4 minutes each day if possible.

Alternate Nostril Breathing

Daily alternate nostril breathing is incredibly beneficial to your well-being. Ancient Yogis, who practiced yoga thousands of years ago, believed that many diseases were connected to irregular nasal breathing. As your nose is directly linked to your brain, alternate nasal breathing allows both sides of the brain to function optimally, which in turn calms the mind. Its other benefits include improving sleep, boosting the pineal gland, balancing hormones, and calming the nervous system.

Simply inhale through the left nostril, while closing the right with your thumb. Hold the breath, covering both nostrils. Release your right nostril and exhale.

Now inhale through your right nostril, again hold the breath covering both nostrils, and then exhale through your left nostril.

This counts as one round: you can either do it slowly in your own time or inhale for the count of 4, hold for 10 and exhale for 8. Try to do 6–10 rounds every day for 21 days and notice the difference.

BREATHING EXERCISES

Breathing to Relax

During times of stress, it is common for us to tighten our chest, grip our shoulders, and shorten our exhalations, even to the point of not exhaling at all so that we are holding our breath.

How to breathe to relax

To enhance relaxed breathing, you need to consciously relax your chest, shoulders, neck, jaw, and tongue. Then imagine the breath easily flowing and filling the deepest parts of your lungs. Bring awareness to your breath. The speed and depth will alternate—just observe this without trying to change a thing. Simply focusing on your breath can create a calm and serene state of being. To achieve this, move your belly with each breath. When you inhale, the diaphragm descends toward your abdomen, which pushes the abdominal muscles and gently swells your belly. As you exhale, the diaphragm releases back toward the heart, enabling the belly to release toward the spine.

For a quick and effective way to relax through a stressful situation, breathe in through your nose, keeping your mouth closed and tongue relaxed, holding for the count of 4, then when you have finished inhaling, hold for the count of 2 and then slowly exhale to the count of 6.

Viparita Karani

Another good exercise for calming is to lie with your bottom against a wall and your legs up the wall at a right angle. To get in this position you will need to sit on the floor facing the wall and maneuver your legs up the wall and wriggle yourself so that your bottom touches the wall. Remain in this position for 15 minutes doing nothing, just sitting with yourself and breathing. This will make you feel centered and filled with contentment.

WE ALL NEED TO BREATHE; OF COURSE IF WE DIDN'T WE WOULD DIE! BECOMING AWARE OF HOW BREATHING CHANGES UNDER DIFFERENT CIRCUMSTANCES AND TEACHING YOURSELF TO BREATHE PROPERLY ARE SOME OF THE MOST SIMPLE, YET BENEFICIAL, THINGS YOU CAN DO FOR YOURSELF. THE AIM OF THESE EXERCISES IS TO KEEP YOU RELAXED AND CALM THROUGH ALL THE UPS AND DOWNS OF LIFE.

Breathing to Sleep

This is a very quick and thorough way of inducing sleep. You start with your relaxation breath, and then expand your breath so that you feel as if you are breathing your awareness into your entire body. As you breathe in, allow the breath to reach every part of your body— beginning with your feet.

How to breathe to sleep

Take your breath and awareness to your toes and feet and silently say to yourself "I relax my toes and feet; my toes and feet are relaxed and happy." Then switch your focus up to your calves and give them your breath and attention. Slowly move your breath and awareness up through your whole body, including all your inner organs, until you are breathing into your head, brain, and the top of your scalp.

Hopefully by this point you will be asleep, but if for any reason you're not, then breathe into your head and as you exhale, imagine all your worries and thoughts releasing through the top of your head.

Breathing to Energize

I recommend you repeat this exercise three times a day as a general strengthener and to sustain energy and good health.

How to breathe to energize

Using deep, hearty breaths here, breathing through the nose again, mouth closed and with your tongue relaxed: breathe in for the count of 2, hold for the count of 4, and breathe out for 2 counts. Repeat this sequence of breaths 10 times.

Breathing to focus the mind

Another exercise I find very helpful if I am feeling anxious is to get into the yoga position known as Downward Facing Dog. To me this exercise is extremely valuable. I use it if I need to be energized, if I'm angry or confused, in fact in any emotional state. It can be incredibly beneficial.

Get onto your hands and knees, setting your knees directly below your hips and your hands slightly forward of your shoulders. Make sure your palms are spread, your fingers parallel or slightly turned out, and your toes are turned under.

Now exhale and lift your knees away from the floor, ensuring your tailbone is lengthened away from the back of your pelvis. Do ten deep breaths, in through your nose, out through your nose, making that Darth Vader sound I described earlier as if you are brushing the back of your throat with your breath.

YOGA

I was first introduced to yoga by my mother when I was 15 because she thought it would help with the breathing difficulties I always had as a child. I took some classes and enjoyed them immensely, but it took me a long time to truly get it and to fully understand what yoga does and what its benefits are. In my mid-teens I was just too restless and unable to concentrate. Many years later after numerous classes, courses, and instructions from some of the best teachers in the world, I feel I can finally incorporate yoga into my daily life without it being a chore and now it brings me only joy and a sense of calm.

Yoga has been practiced for at least 2,500 years when an Indian author named Patanjali wrote the yoga sutras, which constituted the first yoga text known to be written. He defined yoga as *chitta-vritti-nirodhah*, which means the cessation of the turning of the mind. This is exactly what it means to me: a calming of the mind, so that the whirlwind that exists in my head can slow down and stop. The postures physically stretch and tone your body, of course, keeping it young and supple, but the higher aim is to connect with the universe so your mind, body, and soul are all at one. The inner stillness is fantastic.

Yoga does many things for you. It stimulates your glands and cleanses your vital organs. It creates a flexible and strong body, improves respiration, energy, and vitality, helps to maintain a balanced metabolism, promotes cardio and circulatory health, relieves pain, helps you look and feel younger, and improves your athletic performance.

TYPES *of* YOGA

There are many different schools of yoga and I have tried nearly all of them. Your preference really is a personal choice; the end results and benefits are more or less the same.

01

02

03

01 Ashtanga (or Astanga)

Ashtanga is the name given to the system of yoga taught by Sri K. Pattabhi Jois. Physically it is demanding, as it involves synchronizing breathing with a progressive and continuous series of postures. This process produces intense internal heat and a profuse, purifying sweat that detoxifies muscles and organs. The result is improved circulation, flexibility, stamina, and a calm mind. I find Ashtanga can be highly addictive as you zone out completely when practicing the repetitive routines.

02 Dharma Mittra

Dharma Mittra is a very physical sequence that involves a lot of balancing, twisting, stretching, and back bends. It feels quite athletic or contemporary dance based. These sequences are a little different than other types of yoga and are more intense; I recommend you try this if you are advanced at practicing yoga.

03 Hatha

This is the first type of yoga I tried. I always feel that Hatha is the gentlest form of yoga, making it a good one to start with. It uses postures (asanas) and stretches in combination with the breath to develop flexibility and relaxation. There are many styles of Hatha yoga. It brings balance, strength, and calmness.

04

04 Iyengar

This type of yoga is taught by trying to get every pose exactly correct and with complete alignment. Iyengar teachers believe that one day their students will be able to attain perfect poses through constant practice and that, once they have created the balance in the body, it will be reflected in the mind. Iyengar yoga uses a lot of props—blocks, bolsters, chairs, pillows, and straps.

05

05 Jivamukti

Jivamukti is vinyasa-style yoga, meaning alignment of yoga and breath. Practice and classes are physically quite intense. Each class has a theme, which is explored through yoga scripture, chanting, meditation, asana (yoga postures), pranayama, and music. Jivamukti appeals to those who want a good workout and also something to stretch their minds because it includes chanting and philosophizing. Jivamukti classes can be quite diverse in style and more fun than lots of other classes, and almost feel like you're in a rave!

06 Kundalini

The word *kundalini* refers to the coiled energy of the Root chakra, which surrounds the base of the spine. The principle behind Kundalini yoga is that by freeing up this area, we can unleash the unlimited potential that lies within that energy center. Kundalini can be quite intense and challenging and is a more spiritual style of yoga. It focuses on specific breathing techniques that intensify the effects of the poses with the purpose of freeing energy in the lower body and allowing it to move upward.

06

your

DAILY PRACTICE

I try to practice yoga every day for 20–30 minutes, and then maybe one 90-minute lesson a week. By doing just 20 minutes a day you get the benefits without having to squeeze too much time into your schedule.

This is not a specialized yoga book, but I wanted to include the exercises I couldn't do without that help with moods and emotions. Try to find a local yoga class where you can practice regularly. If you can't, try a recommended yoga book or DVD and practice at home.

Surya Namaskara (Sun Salutation)
There are many different types of sun salutations. This is my favorite because it feels dynamic and complete. The continuous flowing builds heat in the body while raising your heart rate. Each pose coordinates with your breath; you inhale to extend and exhale to bend.

01 Stand in Tadasana (see page 137). Make sure your feet are grounded and the weight is distributed evenly. Bring your hands into prayer position at your heart's center and gently close your eyes and start ujjayi breath.

02 Inhale through your nose and stretch your arms out to the side and overhead into Urdhva Hastasana (Upward Salute). Look upward toward the ceiling.

03 As you exhale, fold into Uttanasana (Standing Forward Bend). Make sure your spine is straight (you can bend your knees if you need to). Keep your legs engaged and draw your kneecaps toward you.

04 Inhale and lengthen your spine forward into Ardha Uttanasana (Half Standing Forward Bend). Lift your gaze ahead, then extend and lengthen the spine. Either place the fingertips on the floor or onto your shins.

05 As you exhale, either step or lightly jump back into plank pose. Your hands should be shoulder distance apart and your feet hip distance. Inhale and lengthen.

06 Exhale and lower into Chaturanga Dandasana (Four-limbed Staff Pose). Either keep your legs straight and push back into your heels or bring your knees to the floor.

07 Inhale and bring your chest forward into Urdhva Mukha Svanasana (Upward Facing Dog). Make sure you pull your shoulders back and down and lengthen your collarbones, gaze upward, and lengthen neck.

08 As you exhale, roll over the toes and come into Adho Mukha Svanasana (Downward Facing Dog). Ground through your hands and feet and push your heels toward the floor. Lengthen your spine and stay here for five breaths. Enjoy this moment.

09 Exhale, bend your knees, and look between your hands. As you inhale, either step or lightly hop your feet between your hands, returning to Ardha Uttanasana.

10 Exhale back to Uttanasana.

11 As you inhale, reach your arms out wide to your sides and come to stand, ensuring your back is lengthening. Draw your arms overhead to Urdhva Hastasana and gently bring them back into prayer position at your heart's center. You can either stay here for a few breaths or go straight into the next sun salutation.

0 2

0 1

0 3

0 4

0 5

0 6

0 7

0 8

yoga for

DEPRESSION

Yoga works for depression and sadness because it promotes deep relaxation. This is achieved by the controlled breathing during the physical poses (asanas). The heart rate is reduced, blood pressure is lowered, and respiration eases. These effects in turn reduce anxiety, depression, and anger.

01 Uttanasana (Forward Fold)

B.K.S. Iyengar, the founder of Iyengar yoga, writes about Uttanasana in his book Light on Yoga: *"Any depression felt in the mind is removed if one holds the pose for two minutes or more." You will really benefit from using this standing pose to lift your mood.*

Stand up straight in Tadasana (see page 137). Exhale and bend forward from the hip joints and not the waist. Lengthen your torso, so you can move more freely into the position. With your knees straight or slightly bent, bring your palms or finger tips beside or in front of your feet with your palms to the back of your ankles. Now with your inhalations and exhalations, lift and lengthen your torso and release a little bit more into the forward bend. Here try resting for 2 minutes, then, when you want to come out of this pose, bring your hands back onto your hips. Lengthen your torso and come up in an inhalation to your standing position.

02 Janu Sirsasana (Head-to-knee Forward Bend)

This yoga position is seated. It is a gentle fold that calms the mind. It also stretches the hamstrings and groin, and stimulates the liver and kidneys.

In a seated position make sure your buttocks are lifted (you can use a folded blanket for this). Position your legs straight in front of you. Inhale and bend your right knee, placing your heel toward the perineum. Rest the sole of your right heel against your left thigh with your right knee close to the floor. From here, hinge forward with your hips, lengthening your spine, with your hands on either side of your right foot. Make sure you don't round your back. Keep looking toward your toes and, by hinging at your waist, your head will be close to your right knee. Breathe deeply in this position for 1–3 minutes, then repeat the pose on the opposite side.

03 Bhujangasana (Cobra)
This asana is a backbend that can be done in stages. It expands the chest and gives elasticity to the lungs. The pose resembles the cobra with its hood raised.

Lie on your stomach with your toes flat on the floor and your forehead resting on the ground. Keep your legs close together and your feet and heels lightly touching each other. Place your palms underneath your shoulders, keeping your elbows parallel and close to your torso. Inhale and lift your head, chest, and abdomen while keeping your navel on the floor. Keep breathing with awareness, and try to straighten your arms by arching your back as much as possible. Tilt your head and look up. Make sure your shoulders are away from your ears. When you are ready to come out of the pose, gently lower your abdomen, chest, and head back to the ground.

Sirsasana (Headstand)

Performing a headstand would be a valuable addition to your daily practice. Not only does it have physical benefits, the emotional ones are tremendous. Inverting yourself reverses the action of gravity on your body; it changes any negative emotions and leaves you feeling a lot better about things.

The headstand stimulates the pituitary glands to produce endorphins, which act to block pain and increase self-esteem. Beginners can start by doing a headstand against a wall.

Use a mat to pad your head and forearms. Kneel on the floor. Interlock your fingers together and place your forearms on the floor, elbows at shoulder width. Roll your upper arms slightly outward, pressing your inner wrists into the floor. Place the crown of your head on the floor.

While inhaling, lift your knees off the floor, walking your feet closer to your elbows, heels elevated. Actively lift through the top of your thighs to form an inverted V. Firm your shoulder blades against your back and lift them toward your tailbone so the front torso stays as long as possible (see photo 01). This should help prevent the weight of your shoulders from collapsing onto your neck and head.

Gently lift your legs up into the air, aligning your body into a straight line.

Try to hold the pose for 20 breaths, or practice staying up for a longer period each time and work toward that.

When you are ready to come down, slowly lower your legs and stay in Child's Pose (see photo 02).

0 1

0 2

yoga for

CALMING

Tadasana (Mountain Pose)

If you feel upset or overwrought, you need a pose that helps you stay focused and grounded. An awareness of your feet being connected to the floor is very calming.

This pose is great at strengthening and toning the whole body as well as improving alignment and balance.

Stand straight with your feet together. Spread your toes out wide apart and make sure you distribute your weight evenly over both feet. Using your muscles around your knees and thighs, pull your kneecaps up, move your thighs back, and tuck your tailbone in. Keep your arms straight by your side, palms facing in. Pull back your shoulder blades and lift your chest, keeping your neck and shoulders relaxed. Look straight ahead. Hold for 1–2 minutes.

Be conscious in this pose and don't just relax. Activate every part of your body, from your feet all the way up to your head.

yoga for

ANGER

A twist can be beneficial for wringing out anger because anger is often held in our inner organs, especially the liver. One of its roles is to transform hormones released during negative emotional states, so they can be eliminated from the body. If the liver is not functioning properly, then it is unable to release the hormones. This causes the body to heat up and negative states such as anger are prolonged.

Ardha Matsyendrasana (Half Spinal Twist)
The half spinal twist is very beneficial for both the liver and spleen. When you inhale, you are breathing fresh new life and then letting everything that is stale and old be washed away by the exhalation.

Sit on the floor with your legs straight in front of you. Now bend both your knees and put your feet flat on the floor.

Slide your right foot under your left leg, all the way to the outside of your left hip. Gently lay the right side of your leg on the floor.

Take your left foot and step it over the right leg. Stand it on the floor beside your right hip. Your left knee should be pointing to the ceiling. Exhale and half twist your spine toward your left thigh.

Put your left hand behind you on the floor by your left buttock.

Put your right upper arm on the outside of your left thigh near the knee.

Keep your tailbone lengthened and make sure your left foot stays firmly in contact with the floor.

Turn your head in the direction of the twist, so toward the left.

With every inhalation, lift your chest a little more through the sternum and then twist deeper as you exhale. Stay in this position for about 30 seconds to 1 minute and then repeat on the other side.

Sarvangasana (Basic Shoulder Stand)

This is another pose that is beneficial at reducing stress and getting rid of any feelings of anger. It helps to increase the blood flow to the upper body, especially the neck, shoulders, and head. It has lots of other benefits including relieving allergies, helping with asthma, stimulating your thyroid, and it can also calm your nervous system.

With this exercise you need to be especially precise, and mindful of your back and your neck so that there is no risk of injury.

Lie on the floor with your legs together. Put your arms close to your body, palms facing up. Make sure you press your head onto the floor and your shoulders and arms are rooted.

Exhale and swing your legs over your head lifting your hips. Elongate your body as long as possible and support your hips with your hands. Be aware of your foundation, keeping the weight distributed mainly on the elbows, then your shoulders, and then your head. If you are comfortable and you feel rooted, hold the position for ten breaths. Once you have achieved this, slowly come down, keeping your weight on your hands to protect your back and neck.

IN SOME FORMS OF YOGA, IT IS ADVISED TO USE A ROLLED-UP BLANKET THAT IS PLACED UNDER THE EDGE OF YOUR SHOULDERS AND NOT UNDER YOUR HEAD AND NECK. THIS CREATES MORE SPACE, EASING PRESSURE ON YOUR NECK.

Shavasana (The Corpse Pose)

As the name suggests, this pose requires you to be as still as a corpse. To get the full benefit, you need to clear your mind of any thoughts and breathe deeply. This pose (my favorite!) is amazing at relaxing your entire body.

Lie on your back with your legs slightly apart. Put your arms beside your body with the palms facing upward. Close your eyes and release any tension from your face, making sure your jaw isn't clenched. Start to visualize every part of your body relaxing, beginning with your feet then your legs, organs, arms, and continue up to your head.

You need to spend 5–15 minutes practicing Shavasana so that you fully relax your body.

MEDITATION

Meditation is something I struggled with right from the beginning. I just didn't get it! I really felt that I was kind of faking it and I just didn't understand what it actually achieved. But I persevered and did many courses with different people, from gong meditation (somebody plays on a huge gong to create really positive vibrations that wash through your body and cleanse your mind) to transcendental meditation and many others. There are many kinds of meditation and you have to really find the type that works for you.

Science has now proven that deep relaxation changes the genetic level of our bodies. One Harvard study found the disease-fighting genes increasing in activity after relaxation practices. Relaxation is a state of rest and physical renewal. It boosts your nervous system by activating the parasympathetic nervous system, causing the body to feel more relaxed. You will have improved digestion, better memory, and a stronger immune system, and you will find yourself more emotionally balanced, with lower blood pressure and a reduction in those cancer-causing free radicals. This state also decreases the mental and physical aging process, improves PMS, and decreases the chances of contracting heart disease.

Meditation is a state of thoughtless awareness; it is effortless. The benefits of meditation are endless, and it can be practiced anywhere at any time for free.

There are many styles of meditation practice, and it may take you a few tries at different approaches until you find one that suits you. I would suggest you meditate for 10–20 minutes daily and commit to practicing for 21 days to give yourself the best chance to experience the benefits. Remember, some days will be easier than others but you will still be benefitting.

FOLLOWING
THE BREATH

As the name suggests, this form of meditation focuses on your breath. Make no effort to control the breath, just observe its rhythm with no judgment. Some breaths will be deep, and some shallow. Just concentrate your mind on your breathing: every time you notice yourself in thought, gently bring your attention back to the breath.

Sit upright with your spine straight. You can either kneel, cross your legs, or sit on a chair with your feet on the floor. Place your hands, palms turned upward, on your thighs or knees.

Inhale and exhale, slowly and deeply, three times. Focus on relaxing your body as you breathe out. Your eyes can be open or closed; I prefer to close them.

Then just allow your breath to come in of its own accord: make no attempt to control it. Simply observe your breath, flowing in, and flowing out. If any thoughts come, just notice them and let them go, and return your attention to your breath.

Feel the air flow effortlessly in through your nostrils and into your abdomen. Feel your abdomen rise on the inhalation then fall again as the breath flows out.

Sometimes people like to concentrate on the whole breath, but you may find it easier just to focus on the breath's movement through your nose, or in your abdomen or maybe in your diaphragm, whatever works best for you.

JUST CONCENTRATE YOUR MIND ON YOUR BREATHING: EVERY TIME YOU NOTICE YOURSELF IN THOUGHT, GENTLY BRING YOUR ATTENTION BACK TO YOUR BREATH.

MANTRA MEDITATION

During a mantra meditation, you mentally repeat a calming word, sound or mantra that will take you away from all your busy thoughts. Again your mind will wander and when you notice that it has, just gently bring your attention back to your mantra.

There is no right or wrong way to do this. Just remember to relax and let the mantra effortlessly fill your mind. Some days my mind is so busy that I barely remember to come back to my mantra but even so I still feel and receive the benefits.

You begin in an upright seated position just as you did with the previous meditation exercise.

Inhale and exhale deeply three times. Instead of focusing on the breath, replace the awareness with mentally repeating your mantra.

A few popular mantras are:
Om/aum (it is, will be, to become)
Love
Ham-Sah (a Hindu variant meaning I am he/that)
I am that I am
Om Mani Padme Hum (hail the jewel in the lotus)

Another form of mantra meditation is transcendental meditation, or TM, where the teacher provides you with a mantra. There are many places that teach TM: I can highly recommend the David Lynch Foundation as being very reputable and a good place to learn.

MINDFUL
MEDITATION

During mindful meditation, you expand your awareness of the present moment— your focus is entirely based on what you are experiencing at that point in time.

Mindful meditation can be practiced whether you are sitting or moving around. Your focus could be on a thought, or your breath, or the sensation of your hands on your legs or your feet on the floor. It seems quite simple, but even the act of sitting and focusing on one thing can bring you back into the now and ease you into a light meditation.

Alternatively, you can practice mindful meditation as you go about your everyday business, for example while washing up, cooking, shopping, or walking down the street. The reason this works is we can use these normal daily activities as our focus. We become mindful of our experiences, keeping our awareness involved. I prefer walking meditation, which I use daily while walking to the station on my way to work.

Unlike the other forms of meditation, you keep your eyes open during this meditation. There is a focus and an awareness that sometimes gets ignored if we don't actively practice mindful meditation. This might be the sounds of nature, other people, cars, or machines.

Meditating while your body is in motion seems to be easier for most people compared to when you are sitting still. This is because a lot of people don't have the patience to sit still and you can feel uncomfortable sitting still for a long time.

This meditation can be an intense experience and can also bring enjoyment. As long as you are aware of yourself, you are being mindful. Again there is no need to change anything or to judge. Just observe whatever is happening, your thoughts, feelings, or sensations. It is simply about bringing your attention into the moment, focusing your awareness fully on what you are doing.

CANDLE
MEDITATION

This form of meditation can lead you into an intense meditation that will bring you serenity, calmness, and improve your concentration. In this hypnotic state, the mind settles and you can focus your attention on no topic at all and allow your mind to become completely quiet.

You want your environment to be comfortable before you begin this technique—make sure you are warm and the lights are dimmed.

Place a burning candle that is at eye level when you adopt an upright seated position.

Deeply inhale and exhale three times.

Focus your attention on the candle flame, watching with ease how it flickers. Sit for a while like this and then in your own time close your eyes.

Now focus your attention on your mind's eye or third eye, which is situated on the bridge of your nose between your eyebrows. You will most likely see the imprint and image of the flickering flame in your imagination. If for any reason you don't, reopen your eyes and watch the burning flame until when you close your eyes again you have the image of the flame imprinted in your mind.

Gently observe the image in your mind's eye until it fades away, then open your eyes again and repeat. As before, there is no right or wrong way to do this; it is meant to be relaxing and effortless. Repeat this exercise for 10–20 minutes.

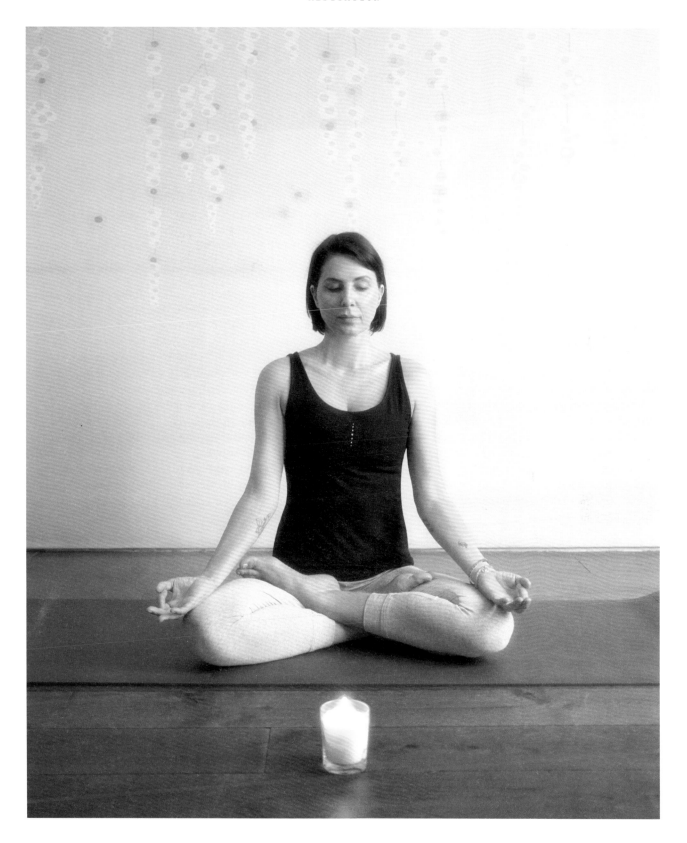

ORGANIZING YOUR DAY

how to keep on track & stay positive

For all of us women, there is a lot to do within a day. We all have very busy lives and we are constantly multitasking. In my case having four kids, three businesses, a need to exercise, run my home, my life, kids' lives, dogs' lives, wanting to eat healthily, and so on … it can all become really stressful. And yes, sometimes my regime completely falls apart. I eat the wrong food, drink too much, and some days I just don't feel motivated to exercise. But nobody is perfect and when you feel like this you just have to draw a line through that day and start again. Well, that's what I do! But we have to keep on going and moderate our lives rather than being judgmental and self-critical.

Through everything you do, you still have to love yourself. I always tell myself that provided I am good 95 percent of the time, for the other 5 percent I can live my life feeling less pressurized and constrained, and that way ultimately I can be happy, as I am not under such scrutiny. After all, it is so important to live life to the full. A friend said to me once, "Sadie, you have got to start living. Stop worrying!" If you start considering how many summers you have left when you will be physically fit enough or adventurous enough to jump off the side of a boat, it gives you the impetus to utilize your time more fully and actually go for it and be daring!

With so much to think about, there are several strategies to help you put yourself under less pressure, not least being organized and managing your time carefully—especially if you have a very full day ahead of you. When I've got a busy day ahead and I know I won't have time to get food, I put a couple of packets of miso soup and a pack of almonds in my handbag for snacking on. Then I won't get hungry and reach for a chocolate bar. And even though making lists and schedules may seem a little clinical, they do help you feel in control and confident that you're getting everything done, which keeps your mind at peace.

I like to try to make the first few hours after I wake as smooth as possible because if that happens then the rest of the day tends to work out too. Preparing

I LIKE TO TRY TO MAKE THE FIRST
FEW HOURS AFTER I WAKE AS SMOOTH
AS POSSIBLE BECAUSE IF THAT
HAPPENS, THEN THE REST OF THE DAY
TENDS TO WORK OUT TOO.

146

breakfast, doing the school run, and getting to work can all become a lot easier if we follow a few simple steps and start the day focused, grounded, and unstressed. Of course, if you can include a walking meditation when you are walking to work, returning from school, or taking your dogs to the park, you ground yourself and start the day positive and calm. While I walk my dogs, I try to think of as many positive thoughts as possible. If a negative thought comes into my mind, I replace it with a positive. The more you do this the more your mind has positive thoughts. Harboring resentments is not good for anyone, so if I am consumed with resentment toward somebody or something, I try my hardest to alleviate this. A friend of mine gave me a tip for times when my mind is full of resentful thoughts about one person or some intense situation. She suggested I visualize shrinking the thought or image in question, turning it into black and white, and sending it to another part of the world. I tried this and it really works; it gives the resentment less importance.

147

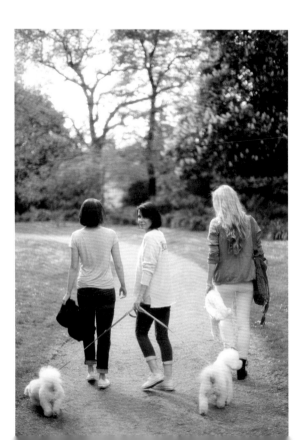

my morning

ROUTINE

I start my day with oil swilling, which is also called oil pulling. I swill a small spoonful of unrefined good-quality oil (I use coconut) all around my mouth, like you would with a mouthwash but with none of the chemicals those products contain. Oil swilling attracts and removes bacteria, toxins, and parasites that live in your mouth or lymph system, and also pulls any congestion and mucus from your throat and loosens up your sinuses. With the help of your saliva, all these unwanted things bind with the oil, ready to be spat out. The process also helps to remineralize your teeth and strengthen your gums by thoroughly cleansing the mouth area.

While I am swilling I do some gentle stretches like the Downward Facing Dog (see page 132) or I kneel in Child's Pose (see page 136) or I just kneel with my big toes together and my bottom on my heels. I exhale and place my forehead on the floor, swilling the whole time. In this position I will take many breaths, breathing into my spine, creating space. After just a few minutes, it is amazing how much my spine has lengthened. Another simple exercise to warm up and extend the spine is to sit cross-legged and rotate from the hips. First clockwise, then reverse circles counterclockwise, 5 one way and 5 the other, with your hands on your knees pressing down, pushing your torso in a circle.

Any of these exercises allows me to create some space in my body, aligning my spine and lengthening my breath. I finish with a short meditation, usually in Lotus Position (Padmasana), which means sitting cross-legged. To perfect this pose, each foot is placed on the opposite thigh, keeping the knee joint as close as possible to the floor while rotating your hip joints.

My routine takes about 20 minutes, which is enough time to swill. Once I have finished the oil swilling, I spit the oil into a tissue and put it in the bin to avoid any issues with blocking toilets or sinks. Then, I swish out my mouth a few times with clean water.

After a night's sleep, your body can become quite acidic. To counteract this I prepare myself a cup of warm water and squeeze the juice of a lemon or half a lemon (or lime) into it; this restores my body to a more alkaline state. Even though lemon tastes very bitter and tart, it is in fact alkaline and not acidic. Another good tip to alkalize the body in the morning is to add a tablespoon of apple cider vinegar to a glass of water. The whole acid/alkaline food topic is very interesting and I try to follow it as closely as I can (see opposite).

GREEN POWER
SMOOTHIE

The last part of my morning routine is to make a power smoothie. This one, invented by my sister Jade, will set you up for the whole day!

There are many opinions about the benefits of juicing and drinking smoothies. My advice is to eat a healthy diet and enjoy juicing and green smoothies from time to time. Substituting juicing and smoothies for meals is not a good idea.

1 banana
1 small package acai pulp
1 handful frozen berries
2 tablespoons protein powder
1 handful spinach or kale
2 teaspoons super green mix
  (spirulina, wheat grass, and
  barley grass)
2½ cups almond milk
1 teaspoon bee pollen

Put everything except the bee pollen into a blender and process for about 45 seconds. Add more almond milk if you prefer a thinner consistency. Pour into a glass and sprinkle the bee pollen on top—it gives the smoothie a lovely little crunch and tastes delicious!

Tips to counter too much acid in the body:

Drink plenty of water—12 cups a day is best. Make sure it is filtered.

Have a big salad once a day, which includes green leafy vegetables such as kale, spinach, broccoli, asparagus, and parsley.

Use black pepper on anything savory.

Snack on pumpkin seeds or add them to salads.

Swap your table salt for Himalayan or sea salt.

Drink ginger tea as it is very alkalizing.

Swap balsamic vinegar for apple cider vinegar.

Squeeze lemon or lime juice on salads or in your herbal teas.

Reduce stress—it plays a big role on the pH of your body and whether it is acidic or alkaline.

FENG SHUI

It doesn't require a lot of effort or investment to organize your home along Feng Shui principles and the benefits can be immediate. You should enjoy bringing positive energy into your home and feel a lot happier and healthier for it.

Steps to Remove Negative Energy

Decluttering removes negative energy and frees space to bring new life and positive forces into your home.

1) Start by opening windows/doors to allow the air to flow freely. Draw back the curtains and let the light shine in.

2) Clear out all your clutter, as this could be blocking your good energy and fortune. Typical areas where we allow clutter to accumulate are behind doors, on tops of wardrobes, and under beds.

3) Give your home a thorough clean from top to bottom. Hopefully, it will be less of a mammoth task now that you have dealt with those junk spots.

4) Sound is a very effective and instant way to clear the energy in any space. Start by walking around your home clapping; this will break up any stagnant or blocked energy, allowing it to flow freely. Alternatively, walk around your home ringing a bell or chanting or singing. Singing clears and uplifts the energy of your home, as does playing music.

Rebalancing Your Home

Feng Shui uses the four elements of Fire, Water, Earth, and Air to bring balance and harmony into a space.

Fire

Fire has been used for purification since ancient times. Churches, mosques, synagogues, and temples all use fire in their religious and sacred rituals. In your home, cleansing with fire is as simple as lighting a candle. Whenever I light a candle I put my intention forward—be it a need to bring peace and well-being or a more specific intention such as to attract a mate or get a job. Then I place it in the appropriate area—for example, if I am having problems with my finances, I place the candle in my Fortunate Blessings Area.

Water

Water is the symbol of harmony. For best results, use water from a natural spring or waterfall, or water from an unpolluted river or stream. Bless the water by holding your hands over the bowl while you either pray or chant, all the while focusing on your intentions. Then use the blessed water to purify your home, sprinkling it wherever you feel inclined. I put the water into a spray bottle and walk around spraying the entire space.

Earth

Salt is a powerful means of purification and is universally renowned for its healing properties. It is also said to absorb negativity. When I space clear, I like to put either a bowl of salt in every room, or a line of salt across every doorway. Leave the salt for 24 hours, by which time it should have absorbed all the negativity.

Air

Burning incense is one of the most readily available and popular ways of purifying the air. You can also burn essential oils in an oil burner.

Electromagnetic Fields

Electromagnetic fields, or EMFs, are environmental pollution. EMFs are the fields created by electrical wiring, satellite dishes, microwaves, televisions, and all the technical devices most of us have in our homes. Ways in which you can reduce the severity of EMFs include turning off all appliances and pulling out the plugs. Placing plants and crystals near or on electrical equipment helps to lessen the EMFs.

Crystals

Crystals are powerful Feng Shui aids that can be placed in an appropriate area of your home to absorb negative energy and promote healing. There are many books and websites on the properties of crystals: rose quartz, for example, is the crystal of love; amethyst is thought to promote peace and tranquility. I place an amethyst crystal under my bed to encourage a peaceful night's sleep.

Crystals that help alleviate and block geopathic and environmental stress are brown jasper, amazonite, amethyst, diamonds (worn as earrings are very effective against the rays that are emitted by mobile phones), fluorite, larimar, obsidian, and smoky quartz. Placing any of these crystals by your computer, microwave, or television, along with plants such as peace lilies, spider plants, and Chinese evergreens can help clear geopathic stress and cleanse the air.

Flowers

Flowers are used for their color and beauty to enhance and uplift any space. They can also be used alongside plants in specific areas to raise the energy levels. Always use fresh flowers and keep the water clear.

EMBRACING FENG SHUI IS A FUN AND POSITIVE EXPERIENCE THAT WILL ALLOW GOOD TO FLOW INTO YOUR LIFE.

HEALTH

&

BEAUTY

For ultimate health and beauty, I believe we should try and have as much of a naturalistic approach as possible. When I see someone radiating both health and beauty from inside and out, it is the most beautiful and simple thing. It is not a daunting or complicated process, but one where you consider different factors and try to look at the whole approach to health rather than just trying to find a cream that will make your skin look better on the outside.

When you see a supple, lean body, it usually shows a person who eats well and moderately and who exercises so they are agile and energized.

In my next section, I give some simple and holistic ideas on hair care, how to achieve glowing skin, how to radiate health, and some simple tips that you can add to your daily routine to make you feel your best. There are some face masks, body soaks, and other treats that I love using when I need that extra bit of nourishment. There are also a few quick tips to add to your daily routine that I have found to be very beneficial and make me feel at my best.

It doesn't have to be complicated, but to have general well-being, health, happiness, and beauty, you need to address it from all areas: your diet, fresh air, fresh, healthy food, body brushing, some form of exercise, lots of water, lots of sleep, and making sure you have peace of mind. If you do all of these you will be able to achieve your optimum in both health and beauty.

love your

SKIN & HAIR

It's entirely possible to spend a small fortune on skin and haircare products, but there are lots of natural ingredients you will have in your home that will do amazing things for your appearance at a fraction of the cost.

Of course, plenty of fresh fruit and vegetables in your daily diet is good for your appearance, but directly applying natural ingredients to your skin and hair will also help. Here are some of my favorite natural remedies that can yield great results:

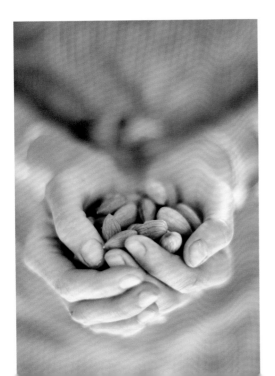

Almond oil

This is an incredible source of vitamins A, B, and E, all of which are great for your skin's health. Almond oil helps to maintain the moisture levels of your skin and gets absorbed really quickly without blocking your pores. It is particularly useful if you have extremely dry, sensitive, or irritated skin.

Avocado

This wonder fruit is rich in monounsaturated oils, which are easily absorbed into the skin. Avocados also contain vitamin E, one of the best ingredients for dry skin, and they plump your skin with lots of moisturizing benefits.

Banana

This tasty fruit contains significant amounts of vitamins C and B6, both of which play vital roles in maintaining the elasticity of the skin, as well as vitamin A. Mashed bananas are a great natural moisturizer that helps repair damaged, dull, and dry skin.

Eggs

Eggs too help with the repair of skin tissue. Egg white is great for generally toning the skin and closing pores and the yolk acts as a natural moisturizer. The lutein contained in egg yolk is immensely good at keeping your skin elastic and hydrated.

Beaten egg makes a great conditioner for dry and brittle hair—just apply it to damp hair, leave for 20 minutes, then rinse off with warm water.

Goat milk

Goat milk contains precious minerals like selenium and is packed full of vitamins, particularly A, the most important vitamin for skin. As with other milks, goat milk contains lactic acid, an alpha-hydroxy acid (AHA) that can gently slough off dead skin cells and help to hydrate and brighten the skin. Goat milk is an extremely useful beauty ingredient because it is rich in essential fatty acids and triglycerides. The pH of those essential fatty acids is similar to that of humans, so it is less likely to irritate and is easily absorbed by your skin.

Honey

This delicious sweetener is another natural moisturizer that works wonders on dry skin. It also has many antiseptic qualities, which can be very beneficial to people with oily skin that is prone to breakouts. Applied directly to the skin, honey leaves a very soft, satiny feel.

Lemon

Lemon juice is a natural antiseptic so it is a great ingredient to apply to your skin and hair. It is a cooling agent that helps with skin problems such as sunburn, insect stings, acne, and eczema. It also acts as an anti-aging remedy and can remove wrinkles by contributing to collagen production.

Lemon juice can also be used on your hair to treat problems like dandruff and acts as a stimulant if you find that your hair is falling out. A tablespoon of lemon juice applied directly to washed, towel-dried hair can give it real shine, and it is great for blonde hair that needs a little boost.

Oats

Oats contain vitamin E, which is one of the antioxidant vitamins that can help counteract the damaging effect of free radicals in the skin. Oats are very soothing, gently exfoliating, and they help to lighten the skin.

Sugar

Sugar is a natural humectant, meaning it absorbs moisture from the environment so, when you apply sugar to your skin, it actually helps to hydrate it and keep moisture within. It is also a natural source of glycolic acid, another alpha-hydroxy acid (AHA) that penetrates the skin and breaks down the "glue" that bonds skin cells, encouraging the cell regeneration that gives you fresher, younger-looking skin. Sugar makes a great exfoliant when added to other ingredients; you can choose granulated, brown, or superfine sugar depending on how deep you want to scrub (see page 156).

FACE MASKS & BODY SCRUBS

Avocado face mask

Avocado is wonderful for adding moisture to tired or dry skin thanks to the vitamin E and monounsaturated oils it contains.

Simply mash the flesh of 1 ripe avocado in a bowl and apply to your face and neck. Leave for 30 minutes and then wipe off using cotton pads dipped in warm water.

For combination skin
Simply add 1 beaten egg yolk to the mashed avocado. Apply to the face and leave for 30 minutes, then remove with damp cotton pads.

For tired, aging skin
Add 1 tablespoon of honey and 1 beaten egg yolk to the mashed avocado and mix to a smooth creamy texture. Apply to the face and leave for 30 minutes, then remove with damp cotton pads.

Honey and banana face mask

Try using this if your skin feels dehydrated—honey and banana are both extremely moisturizing.

Mash 1 small ripe banana in a bowl until it's a smooth creamy paste. Stir in 1 tablespoon oatmeal and 1 teaspoon of honey. Apply to the face and leave for 15–20 minutes, then remove with damp cotton pads.

Lemon cleanser

Lemon juice acts as an antibacterial agent, so it will help with oily skin, breakouts, and also balances the pH of the skin. The egg white tightens and tones the skin.

Mix together 1 teaspoon of freshly squeezed lemon juice and 1 stiffly beaten egg white and apply to your face. Leave for about 10 minutes and then wash off in warm water or with rose water.

Sugar scrub

Sugar has an antibacterial as well as an exfoliating effect on the skin, so this scrub is really beneficial for oily or spotty skin. Choose from superfine, granulated, or brown sugar, depending on how deep you want to scrub. I recommend brown or granulated for the body and superfine sugar for the face and neck.

Mix 1 teaspoon sugar with a few drops of hot water in your hands and gently massage into your skin. Rinse off with cool water and pat dry with a towel.

Coconut and rose body scrub

Try using this scrub on your body while you're waiting for your bath to fill up. It works so well at exfoliating and hydrating skin. Soothing coconut oil combined with sugar will scrape off dead skin cells and clean blocked pores without irritating your skin. The oil will leave the skin soft, even, and help close your pores. The sugar is antibacterial, so great for dealing with breakouts.

⅓ **cup coconut oil**
⅓ **cup granulated sugar**
10 drops rose essential oil

Mix the ingredients together in a bowl. Take some of the mixture and gently rub over your body, paying particular attention to any hard areas of skin on your elbows, knees, and heels. Once you have rubbed it all over, get into your bath and rinse it off. The coconut oil and sugar will dissolve into the bath and make it smell amazing! Soak for as long as you like.

BATH SOAKS

Retreating to a warm bath can work miracles on skin problems, aching joints, and sore muscles and is generally therapeutic after a hectic or stressful day. Adding everyday ingredients such as sea salt and tea or essential oils such as lavender or rose to the water will soothe specific ailments.

Detox bath

Try this soak to help with skin irritations, boost your magnesium levels, or for a great detoxifying bath after a stressful day at work.

¼ cup sea salt or Himalayan salt
¼ cup Epsom salts
¼ cup baking soda
⅓ cup apple cider vinegar
10 drops essential oil, e.g.
   lavender, peppermint, rose

Put the salts and baking soda into a heatproof pitcher. Add ⅔ cup of boiling water and allow the salts to dissolve. Fill the bath with warm/hot water and add the apple cider vinegar and the essential oils. Lastly add the salts to the bath.

Soak in the bath for about 30 minutes. This is a detoxifying bath and you may feel light-headed when you get out, so do be careful.

Milky bath

This bath soak leaves your skin feeling silky smooth due to the lactic acid in the milk, which hydrates the skin and helps with exfoliation.

Warm 2 cups goat milk in a pan and add to your hot bath. Soak in the bath for around 20–30 minutes. You can add 10 drops of your favorite essential oil to help you relax even more.

A bath full of tea!

This bath soak is so easy to do. Simply brew 3–4 large cups of strong hot tea and add them to your bath. Try different types of teas for different effects. Here are a few of my personal favorites to choose from, but feel free to experiment with any tea you like:

English breakfast tea
This is good for itchy skin, since the blend contains high levels of tannins that have both anti-inflammatory and antiviral effects.

Chamomile tea
Chamomile has a calming effect on the body, so this is a relaxing and soothing bath. Perfect at bedtime, it is also beneficial for skin conditions like eczema and chicken pox, common swellings, or infection.

Green tea
The B vitamins in green tea can make you feel happier and lift your spirits, leaving you feeling uplifted and energized. Green tea is also full of antioxidants polyphenols, theanine, and tannin that have powerful effects on the body, soothing sore muscles, open wounds, rashes, cold sores, and many more.

FACE & NECK
EXERCISES

It's so important to keep the facial muscles toned and supple. Facial exercises keep your skin looking younger and help reduce lines. All of these can be done when you're waiting for a bus, you've stopped at a red light, or are walking in the park.

Skin can be very forgiving. Of course you can't reverse the aging process completely, but by stimulating blood circulation you can tighten and tone the natural contours of your face. We go to the gym and work out our bodies, so why not do the same for our faces? With regular exercises, you will see a big change, so give it a try.

Eyes

Our eyes can be one of the first places to show signs of aging. To keep them toned and reduce sagging muscles and crow's feet, try these yoga facial exercises. They will also strengthen your eyes.

Take a deep breath in and keep your head in its normal position. Without moving your head, look up as high as you can. Hold the pose for 5–10 seconds.

Now look downward and hold for 5–10 seconds.

Look up to the top right corner and hold this pose for 5–10 seconds.

Next, look up to the top left corner and hold for 5–10 seconds.

Then start rotating your eyes in a clockwise motion, trying to look as far as you can to the corners, top and bottom. Do this a few times and then repeat in a counterclockwise direction.

BY STIMULATING BLOOD CIRCULATION,
YOU CAN TIGHTEN AND TONE THE NATURAL
CONTOURS OF YOUR FACE.

Mouth

We use our mouths to eat, drink, talk, sing, and smile. With time they can lose tone and start to droop at the corners, making us look unhappy. By doing the exercises below you will strengthen the muscles around your lips and prevent drooping. Do these exercises every day to put the smile back on your face!

Pretend you are kissing the air: pucker your lips as tightly as you can and blow 10 kisses.

With your mouth closed, use your tongue to feel all around the outside of your top teeth. Start with the molars at the back and move your tongue all the way to the other side and then repeat with the bottom teeth. Keep moving your tongue around in this circular movement and then go the other way. Do this 10–15 times.

Keeping your lips together, blow out the right cheek to make a balloon shape and hold for a few seconds. Then do the same with your left cheek and repeat 20 times. Finally, blow out both cheeks at the same time and slowly release the air. This works on reducing laughter lines by toning the facial muscles around this area.

Use your thumbs and index fingers to hold your upper lip. Your thumbnail should touch the upper gums. Totally relax and gently pull your lip downward. Move along the whole lip and repeat 5 times. This will help with any lines across the top of the lip.

Forehead

We use our forehead for lots of expressions and, with time, lines begin to appear, especially if we frown a lot! By releasing the tension in these muscles, we create better blood flow and allow the muscles to relax and go back to their normal position.

To get rid of these lines, use your fingertips to make circular movements around the top of your scalp. Reducing tension here helps the forehead. Do this for a couple of minutes.

Take the palm of your hand and press it against your forehead. Keeping your hand in that position, try to move your head downward. This will pull your forehead up and act as a lifting technique. Repeat this process 5 times.

Place your thumbs on your temples and both index fingers in the center of the top of your forehead. Pull upward and you should feel your whole forehead lifting upward. Hold it for 5 seconds and then repeat the action 5–10 times.

Eyebrows

These exercises release the tension around the eyebrows and are really good at easing tension and headaches. They help to reduce frown lines and give the eyes a more lifted appearance.

Put your thumbs on either side of the top of your nose where your eyebrows start. Using your index fingers and thumbs, pinch the fleshy part around the eyebrows and use circular movements all the way along to massage and release the muscle. You can increase the pressure a little bit each time.

Sweep your index fingers along the eyebrows starting from the bridge of your nose and ending at your temples. You can increase the pressure each time—it should feel like a big release of pressure.

Neck

The skin around our necks is very fine and is one of the first places where we notice signs of aging. These techniques will really help to strengthen the muscles of your jaw as well as the platysma, the band of muscle that surrounds your collarbone and upper chest.

Lift your head upward, looking at the sky, to lengthen your neck. Using the back of both hands, sweep upward from the bottom of your neck all the way to the chin. Continue the action for 30 seconds.

Tensing all the muscles in your neck, slowly move your head from right to left. Repeat 10 times, alternating the direction each time. This will tone all the muscles in your neck and stop the skin from sagging.

Look straight ahead and tense all the muscles in your neck. Keep looking at the same point and stick your neck forward but not downward, then bring it back to the normal position. Repeat 10 times.

To finish

Place your index fingers on either side of the bridge of your nose and make small circular movements to the bottom of your nose around your nostrils. This especially helps to clear nasal congestion and aids lymphatic drainage.

Using your thumbs and index fingers, pinch and pluck the skin all over your face. This increases the blood flow and circulation to the face and is the perfect way to end the exercises.

BODY BRUSHING

I couldn't live without...

REFLEXOLOGY

Body brushing has really done wonders for me; since I have been doing it every day, I have seen huge benefits. The tone of my skin has changed, muscle definition has increased, cellulite has disappeared, my metabolism has improved, and I literally feel more alive. It can be done on dry or wet skin, either just before you shower or while you are in it. Body brushing on dry skin has been shown to be better.

Body brushes are widely available at many health stores. They typically have short, firm bristles—look for one made with natural, not synthetic bristles, and a long handle to make it easy to brush your whole body. Body brushing works in a number of ways, and done on a daily basis can provide a number of benefits. By improving vascular blood circulation and lymph drainage, it encourages the discharge of metabolic waste, hence the body can run more effectively. It helps with the nervous system by stimulating the nerve endings so they work better. It also stimulates hormones and increases the absorption of nutrients by eliminating clogged pores. It firms the skin and helps shift cellulite, which is a toxic material that accumulates in fat cells.

Start body brushing first thing in the morning before you take a shower. I prefer to brush in a warm shower on wet skin. I brush for 5–10 minutes and afterward take a cold shower. I strongly advise you to do this—you will notice such a difference. Take your brush and (gently at first) brush in long strokes starting from your feet and always working upward toward your heart. Once you have brushed all the way up to your shoulders, start brushing from your hands toward your shoulders with long sweeping strokes. Overlap the strokes and repeat over the same section 2–3 times. Don't brush over any broken skin or sensitive areas.

Reflexology makes you feel calm and grounded and improves many ailments you may have, including headaches, digestive problems, insomnia, and stress. It works by stimulating, massaging, and applying pressure to different points in your feet or hands (or sometimes ears) in order to stimulate energy flow through the body and promote self-healing.

Reflexologists believe that the body is divided into ten vertical zones or channels, five on the left and five on the right. Each zone runs from the head down to the reflex areas on the feet and hands. By applying pressure to these reflex points, you can stimulate the energy flow through the corresponding body part and release an energy block in any part of the zone. It brings about a deep relaxation and can help return the body to its natural state.

REFLEXOLOGY
WORKS BY
STIMULATING
ENERGY FLOW
THROUGH THE
BODY TO PROMOTE
SELF-HEALING.

DAILY VITAMINS
& OTHER SUPPLEMENTS

I have never really taken a daily vitamin regularly or consistently. I felt that with a good diet that included juices, smoothies, lots of dark vegetables, garlic, olive oil, lemon, ginger, chile, and herbs, I would be ticking all the boxes on the recommended guidelines. Plus, by constantly reminding myself to keep my body alkalized, I felt I should be in good shape. In fact, when I had a blood test recently, I had no deficiency in anything apart from omega 3, which is probably because I do not eat meat or fish, even though I make up for this by ensuring I get plenty of protein from non-animal sources such as tofu, lentils, tempeh, and beans. Even sticking to a good diet, though, it's hard to be completely sure that we have all the vitamins and minerals we need for full health, so I have listed the supplements I would advise you to keep in your fridge: vitamin C, vitamin D, magnesium, probiotics, and omegas 3 and 6.

VITAMINS

to be or not to be?

Vitamin C

Vitamin C, also called ascorbic acid, is a water-soluble nutrient found in some foods. In the body it acts as an antioxidant, protecting cells from the damage caused by free radicals. Free radicals are compounds formed when our bodies convert food we consume into energy. We are also exposed to free radicals every day by things such as cigarette smoke, air pollution, and ultraviolet light from the sun.

Our bodies need vitamin C to make collagen, a protein that is required to help wounds heal. It also helps the immune system work properly and protects the body from disease. Vitamin C can also improve your body's ability to absorb iron.

Vitamin D

Vitamin D is important for growth, good health, and strong bones. The main reason for taking vitamin D is to aid the absorption of calcium and phosphorus, because they are what keep our bones strong.

Most of our vitamin D comes from exposure to sunlight during the summer months—the vitamin is made by our body in reaction to the sunlight. During winter months, people living in temperate climates can lack vitamin D, because they don't get enough sunlight to the skin. Make no mistake, though—sunbathing shouldn't provide our dose of vitamin D: too much exposure to the sun can cause sunburn, premature aging of the skin, and may lead to skin cancer. So make sure your exposure to the sun is for just 10–15 minutes. The best time of day for absorbing vitamin D is between 11am and 3pm.

In winter months, when sun exposure is hard to get, I advise you to take a supplement. Ask your local pharmacy which one they recommend.

Foods rich in vitamin C:
Broccoli, Brussels Sprouts, Cauliflower, Kale, Lemon Juice, Oranges, Papaya, Parsley, Red and Green Bell Peppers, Strawberries, Tomatoes

Foods rich in vitamin D:
Eggs, Mackerel, Sardines

Foods rich in magnesium:
Avocado, Fish, Garlic, Green Leafy Vegetables, Nuts (especially almonds), Parsley, Whole Grains such as Brown Rice, Buckwheat, Barley

Magnesium

Magnesium is essential to the maintenance of healthy bones and teeth because it is needed for the release of calcitonin, the hormone that encourages calcium to be deposited into the bones. Magnesium offers lots of other health benefits, which include transmission of nerve impulses, body temperature regulation, detoxification, and energy production. It can also help with migraines, insomnia, and depression. Taking magnesium supplements has been found to help with panic attacks, stress, anxiety, and agitations. Magnesium is such an important mineral that we need to make sure that we get our daily dose. Sixty percent of magnesium in the body is within our bones and 26 percent is in our muscles, the remainder being soft tissue and body fluids.

Apart from taking supplements to ensure you are getting enough, I have found that soaking in a magnesium salt bath works wonders. You can purchase magnesium and other supplements either online or in many health stores. Magnesium is absorbed through the skin while you bathe, and this is a great way to speed up recovery after a workout. The magnesium helps to produce serotonin, a mood-elevating chemical within the brain that creates a feeling of calm. Magnesium can also reduce irritability by lowering the effects of adrenaline. It can create a relaxed feeling, improve sleep and concentration, and help muscles and nerves to function properly.

Try to limit your intake of coffee, salt, sugar, and alcohol as they increase the excretion of magnesium through urine, thus depleting the magnesium stored in your body.

PH LEVELS

I think it is very important to look at your acid and alkaline imbalance, and you can do this by buying some pH strips and following the instructions. These strips, which can be ordered online, will give you a clear indication of where your body is on the acid and alkaline scale and how it changes throughout the day. An imbalance in your pH can cause minor ailments and more serious ones can develop later if not corrected. Among these are cardiovascular damage, poor immune system, joint pains, osteoporosis, hormone concerns, and premature aging.

There are some very simple steps you can take to balance your pH levels and moderate them so you are keeping your body mainly alkalized. Our bodies have to keep the pH of our blood, cells, and other fluid at just slightly alkaline (pH 7.365). What happens when we eat a diet high in acidic foods such as soda, chocolate, chips, etc., is that the body has to draw upon its own store of alkaline buffers to neutralize the acid-forming effects of our diet. As an example, if we eat a very acidic diet, then our bodies need more calcium from the body, which can lead to osteoporosis. By eating foods that are alkaline, we don't have to draw on supplies within our bodies and we will be much healthier.

One of the things you can do to counter too much acid in the body is to drink lots of water. I always drink hot water and lemon first thing in the morning.

Alkaline foods and drinks:
Asparagus, Broccoli, Garlic, Grapefruit, Herbal Tea, Lemon, Lemon Water, Lime, Mango, Olive Oil, Onion, Papaya, Parsley, Raw Spinach, Vegetable Juices, Watermelon

Foods and drinks that should definitely be avoided:
Beef, Beer, Cheese, Chocolate, Coffee, Ice Cream, Pasta, Pastries, Pork, Shellfish, Soft Drinks, Sugar (white or brown), Wheat, White Flour, White Rice

PROBIOTICS
& OMEGAS

Probiotics

Probiotics are microorganisms such as bacteria or yeasts that are believed to improve health. The digestive system is home to more than 500 different types of bacteria or microflora that help to keep our intestines healthy, assist in digestion, and maintain a strong immune system. If we take a course of antibiotics or we get an infection in the body, the balance of friendly bacteria in our gut can become disturbed. Taking probiotics can improve the function of the intestines and may also help fight bacteria that causes diarrhea.

Natural yogurt contains probiotics, or you can buy supplements from your local health store. I really strongly advise you take these to keep your digestion healthy and boost your immune system.

Omegas 3 & 6

Omegas are essential for brain function, vision, learning ability, mood, and coordination. Having the correct level of omegas may prevent and control a number of inflammatory conditions such as heart disease, arthritis, and immune dysfunction (e.g. asthma and eczema).

There are good levels of omega 3 in:
Flax, Hemp, Pumpkin, Walnut

Omega 6 occur in:
Safflower, Sesame, Sunflower, Corn

I take a vegetarian supplement called blue algae, but you could also take fish oil to ensure you get your omegas. Ask in a health store which one they recommend.

WELL-WOMAN

It is very important to look after every aspect of yourself, from your diet to your body, mind, and soul! I have done as much self-care as I can, but I have also had a lot of help from teachers, natural healers, and conventional doctors.

Check-ups

I have always been very proactive about my health, which includes having regular check-ups, pelvic exams, blood tests, keeping up-to-date and familiar with my breast care, dental visits, and observing the changes in my skin, such as sun damage and moles. By implementing these medical checks regularly, you stay on top of your health and wellness, so if any problems do arise you can immediately take action. As a young woman I had many scares and problems relating to the health of my breasts and pelvic area. This led me to have thorough and regular screening: scans, mammograms, cervix and uterus care, and regular smears to detect pre-cancerous cells, among other things. These checks have probably helped save my life, so that correct treatment could be carried out without delay.

I was lucky enough to be under the care of the medical pioneer Yehudi Gordon, who was a gynecologist at Viveka, a women's health care practice in north London that, sadly, is no longer there. Yehudi has advised and acted as consultant for me for 25 years from early womanhood to being a mature woman with four kids. He has taught me a great deal both spiritually and physically, and I owe an awful lot to him. So if there's any advice that you should take from me, it is to make sure you keep up to date with all your medical checks.

From menstruation to menopause, every stage in a woman's life can be delicate, sensitive, and different. Hormones can control so much of our lives both emotionally and physically, and so to get a better understanding of this I recommend you read up in detail more about these topics. I highly recommend *The Good Birth Companion* by Yehudi Gordon and Nicole Croft, *Birth and Beyond* by Yehudi Gordon, and *The Natural Health Bible for Women* by Dr. Marilyn Glenville.

Pelvic checks

The CDC recommends that women between the ages of 21 and 64 years have a Pap smear (cervical screening/pelvic check) every three years. Cervical screening is used to check the cells in the cervix (neck of the womb) for any abnormalities that could lead to cancer. It is important to also look out for unusual symptoms. If you have any of the following, it is best to speak to a doctor immediately: painful intercourse, an odd-smelling discharge, persistent pelvic pain or unexpected bleeding, unusual dryness, or an increased amount of discharge.

Breast self-exams

Check your own breasts at home every month. Visit the NIH website, which gives a great explanation of how to do this. It is important to check your breasts every month and if anything feels worrying, see your doctor. It is better to be safe, and if breast cancer is diagnosed, the sooner it is treated the better the chance of success.

You need to see a doctor right away if you notice any of the following: a change in size and shape of your breast, especially if you notice this when you move your arm or lift your breast, a rash around your nipple, a red moist area on your nipple that won't heal easily, discharge from your nipple that is not milky, bleeding from your nipple, any pain or discomfort in your breasts or arm pit that won't go away, a new lump on one breast that is not in the same place as the opposite breast, or if your skin looks or feels different, for example dimpling or puckering.

Blood tests

There are a number of blood tests that can be done to assess your general health, and to check how well organs such as the liver and kidneys are functioning. Blood tests just take a few minutes and can be done by a nurse at your doctor's office or local hospital. It is a good idea to have them done every year, especially as you get older.

Urine tests

They are very useful for detecting problems with the kidneys and urinary tract system, diabetes, and bladder cancer. If you notice any blood in your urine, tell your doctor immediately.

Sexual health

The best way to keep yourself safe from infections or passing any on is by using a condom. Get tested for sexually transmitted diseases before you start any new relationship. Many health clinics can test for HIV, chlamydia, herpes, syphilis, and gonorrhea.

Diabetes

If there is a history of diabetes in your family or your BMI is greater than 25, you should get your hemoglobin A1c checked. The Hemoglobin A1c Test gives you an average blood sugar level over the last three months rather than just at one point in time.

Blood pressure

It is really important to get this checked regularly, because high blood pressure can put a strain on your arteries and heart, which means you will be more likely to suffer a stroke, heart attack, or kidney disease. Get your blood pressure checked at least once a year. If it has been abnormally high or low, then you need to check it more frequently.

Cholesterol check

Cholesterol is a fat that is carried around in our bodies and exists in all our cell membranes. Eighty percent of cholesterol is produced by the liver and 20 percent is directly derived from the food we eat. If your cholesterol is too high, it can block the arteries and increase your risk of heart disease and strokes. Make sure you get tested every three to five years.

Eye tests

Regular eye tests are very important because your eyes don't usually hurt if something is wrong. Optometrists can detect the early signs of certain eye conditions before you are even aware of symptoms. You might need glasses for the first time or you may need a different prescription for the glasses you already have. They can also pick up on early signs of diabetes, glaucoma, and macular degeneration. So do have your eyes tested every two years, or more frequently if it has been advised by your doctor.

Dentist

Brush your teeth with fluoride toothpaste twice a day. Floss your teeth daily and remember that smoking, sugary drinks, and sugary food will affect the health of your teeth and gums. So the healthier you are, the longer your teeth will last. Go for a check-up once a year, but if you are prone to tooth decay, then it is suggested to visit every six months.

Skin checks and moles

Look for changes in your skin and moles monthly and get a yearly skin check from your doctor. If you notice any changes to your moles—in color, size, if they are itchy, bleeding, or they have an irregular shape—then you must see your doctor immediately.

Pregnancy, babies, and being a mommy

Pregnancy can be a wonderful thing in a woman's life, a time full of excitement and wonderment. I experienced it four times and all my pregnancies were completely different. I suffered from hyperemesis, a complication that causes vomiting, nausea, and dehydration. I was hospitalized and put on a hydration drip until my body had recuperated and was rested. Also, three out of my four babies were born at 32/33 weeks, which meant their first few hours or days were spent in an incubator. So, even though having my children is the most wonderful thing I have done in my life, I know pregnancy and childbirth can also be complicated and stressful.

I took a natural approach to my pregnancies and to the births, but in no way would I judge the different choices women make: every woman is different, as is every pregnancy. What worked for me, though, was sticking to yoga, reflexology, positive thinking, and visualization as well as meditation, all of which are discussed in this book. These different therapies helped me with my pregnancies and the actual labor (I opted for water births). I tried to eat healthily and stick to my normal diet as much as possible, never giving myself a hard time if I craved only sweets and jelly beans because when you are struggling with morning sickness, you have to, to some extent, follow your cravings.

Beautiful baby

Motherhood is like nothing else. The love you feel is beyond your expectations, and when you see your beautiful innocent child, suddenly your life makes sense. The first few nights after I took my baby home and got to know this new human being were, to me, what dreams are made of. Of course motherhood is tiring and stressful; you have to learn on your feet how to parent your child all the way from being a defenseless little baby to adulthood—mostly without any training. So a lot of it must be instinctive to you and again a very personal thing.

Being a mommy

When my children were born, I chose to co-sleep. I also chose not to let them cry themselves to sleep, and I never ignored them when they were crying and wanted something. Yes, it did mean parenting was really hard, since I had to attend to their every need and be very hands-on. But as with any stage in life, you just get through it and face problems head on. There are highs and lows and I experienced both, including lows when I suffered from severe postpartum depression and was even hospitalized on some occasions. It was over 11 years ago when I suffered from postpartum depression, and at that time there were quite a few stigmas attached to the condition. Many people don't understand the fear and anxiety that accompanies PPD, and think that you should just be happy and not complain that you have a beautiful baby in your arms. The simplest way I can describe it is to say that there is no rationale behind it; it hits you hard and you may experience some of the darkest and scariest days of your life, feeling cut off, lonely, and possibly unsupported. If you have any concerns that you may have postpartum depression, please see your doctor immediately and be reassured there is treatment that will make you feel better. In time, the feelings you have will pass and you will be able to get on with your life.

Motherhood has many different phases, from the cooing baby, the questioning and curious infant, the energetic toddler, to the rebellious and sometimes worrying teenager. You have to evolve with them and try your best to give them unconditional love. I have in no way been the perfect mother and have made many mistakes as we all have. But I have loved my children constantly and tried not to judge and expect unrealistic things from them. To me, being a mother involves teaching my children about the good things in life, being compassionate, generous, and forgiving but also accepting that, at the end of the day, they have to find their own way and learn by their own mistakes—

especially in their teenage years when they find you highly embarrassing and do not listen to a word you say. Above all, I try to stress to my children to have no judgment and to be loyal and loving to themselves.

Family matters and therapy

What is a normal family? What family has a completely normal set-up these days? It is sad but true—what family has not suffered some tragedy, misfortune, or scandal? Life is complicated, painful, but, without sounding too much like a hippy, we are on a journey, experiencing life on life's terms and learning lessons every day.

The dynamics of each family are different and can be constantly evolving. Sometimes we can get into unhealthy patterns, so it can be helpful to get some extra help from someone who is experienced, like a therapist. Whether you are facing things on your own or with a partner or even the whole family, problems can be shifted, aired, and then hopefully remedied.

I have used therapy during various points in my life—when I lost my father, when I was going through a painful break-up, and when I had postpartum depression. Looking back, I can say now that with the work I put into my therapy, my whole life seems less complicated and a whole lot better.

Joint custody and step-parenting

Separation, divorce, joint custody of children, plus step-parenting are becoming an increasingly common part of the modern family. Very few separations are easy and they bring turmoil, change, and sometimes a lot of pain. It is a highly transitional period and requires a long time for everyone to adjust. Both adults and children have a lot of changes to deal with; everything becomes a very different world. There can be a lot of tears and fights, but also the possibility of new and fresh beginnings, which in the long run will make everyone happier.

Then divorce may come, which can be incredibly stressful and destructive. Sometimes it becomes a mini personal war in which no one is the winner apart from the lawyers. Try your hardest to resist petty arguments and mind games, and if you see yourself becoming bitter and negative, surround yourself as well as the person you are having problems with white light. This will create better vibes between you and create a more karmic situation. It can be quite challenging if you have to separate and divorce, dividing your time and splitting up your family. At first your family doesn't feel like your family. It is such a loss and time of grieving when you see your child/children less because it is your ex's turn. I had to throw myself into lots of different things such as hobbies and work hard at keeping an exciting social life including meeting new people. I took up rock climbing, trapeze, script writing, and started new businesses, which was all quite exhausting but also liberating.

Another area we are not prepared for is that of being a step-parent. With the little experience I have had, you should be open, generous, kind, delicate, and never push. Children will always pick up on it if an adult is pushing too hard and not being genuine. So make sure you are not demanding and that you are instinctive and not trying to buy their affection through presents.

No judgment

Judgment can be a very destructive trait. Either to judge yourself or to judge others will only give you inner angst and conflict. So when you notice yourself being critical or having judgmental thoughts about others, try to correct yourself: what works for me is if I tell myself to mind my own business—I immediately stop. Or, if I am beating myself up and judging myself, I think "would I be so hard on someone I love so much, like my daughter?" I must love myself as much as one of my loved ones and stop having negative thoughts about myself—that too will only create negative situations.

Positivity

Always try and make every situation as positive as possible. Be as positive as you can and try to have positive thoughts. By doing this, your life will be more content and peaceful.

Conclusion

There is a certain love and care that we should all give ourselves daily. There are many traps we can all fall into, but there is a way to make things easier and more fun, so you can live a life of contentment. We all try to practice what we preach, but if for some reason things become a little unmanageable and we develop some bad habits, we have to draw a line through it and start again! I hope our book has given some insight into healthy food, exercise, and life in general.

Protect your mind, body, and soul and love yourself and your neighbor.

FIT WOMAN

Holly

I have spent many years as a personal trainer and lifestyle coach to hundreds of people. Some are ordinary women and men wanting to be fitter, some are postnatal women who want to feel body-confident again, some are actors preparing for film roles, and some are people who want to change their bad habits. I've individually tailored each program, but the fundamental principle is the same: discover a healthy lifestyle, and fall in love with exercise.

I'm not talking quick fixes here—there is no secret powder or magic smoothie. I'm talking about long-lasting, maintainable changes that come from a holistic reboot of bad habits.

By sharing my passion and knowledge of fitness and nutrition, I have given my clients the confidence they need to pursue a healthy and active lifestyle. Small changes lead to big differences in terms of happiness, confidence, and weight loss. Learn better habits, and break the bad ones. Most importantly, I teach my clients how to make it all last.

The fundamental principle is the same: discover a healthy lifestyle, and fall in love with exercise.

I was brought up vegetarian and from the age of six I lived in the countryside. We had a massive vegetable garden, so I was introduced to a delicious variety of fresh, seasonal vegetables and had hands-on experience of planting and picking homegrown produce. Watching your food grow from seed and knowing where it has come from helps you appreciate it. I have wonderful memories of podding fresh peas in the summer and digging up the first of the new potatoes, washing off the dirt, watching them boil, and then popping those sweet, delicious, buttery spuds into my mouth. Heaven.

But "vegetarian" does not equal "healthy," and being vegetarian does not automatically imply you follow a varied and healthy diet. When I left home for London, convenience drove my diet and things changed. I replaced all the fresh seasonal vegetables with french fries, frozen dinners, and easy pasta dishes. It was a slippery slope; my tastes began to gravitate to sweet and sugary foods. As a young actress, I found myself out socializing an awful lot and began to smoke and drink too much.

I suffered from colds and coughs all the time and began to feel sluggish, bloated, and low in energy. Eating left me with a horrible stuffed feeling. At 25, I knew I was out of balance.

I was active, yet far from healthy, and was not happy. I started trying different diets—the cabbage soup diet being particularly dissatisfying. I would feel good for a week or so but couldn't sustain the discipline of such extreme diets so I would revert back to bingeing on chocolate (I have always had a sweet tooth) and fall back into my unhealthy habits. This cycle needed to change.

I began reading many healthy eating books. I found them interesting and inspiring and, the more I learned, the more things began to fall into place. It didn't happen overnight. Bad habits often tend to become ingrained much faster than good ones. But slowly I started to make changes—lasting changes. I learned about raw food, food combining, juice fasting, GI (glycemic index), and toxic foods. I took cooking and nutrition classes, which made me realize that I wanted to become a personal trainer. Something very profound happened. In correcting my own bad habits I realized the joy and deep satisfaction it can provide, and I needed to share it.

I finally made the connection between food with no nutritional value and the fact that I was feeling sluggish and getting ill. After countless hours and years of work, the two key things that helped me find the balance I was missing were having the knowledge to know what to eat and how to work out, and understanding how to use it to make it part of my everyday routine. The more I learned about what I was eating and drinking and the long-term effect it was having on my body and overall health, the less I wanted to pollute myself. Today, I make the choice to eat healthy food because it makes me feel good from the inside out. When I eat a nutritious, freshly cooked meal, I feel happy. It's that simple. Drinking hot water with fresh lemon in the morning means I start the day feeling energized. I don't give in to guilt when I occasionally eat dark chocolate or have a glass of wine because overall I know my diet is healthy and balanced.

I have always been active. As a child I climbed trees, ran through fields, and jumped on my trampoline in the garden. When I moved to London at 17, I joined a gym and started practicing yoga (my sister Sadie took me to my first class). In the spirit of balance I sought a high-energy alternative to yoga and soon became hooked on kickboxing. Motivation to exercise has always been easy for me, and just like jumping on my trampoline, it's

because I have chosen things I love to do. I have never considered staying fit to be a chore. When you see kids constantly moving, jumping, skipping, running—they are doing it because it's fun, and they're loving every minute of it.

If I don't like a particular form of exercise, I won't do it—there's another one that I do like. Trying new teachers, new places to train, and new people to train with is all part of the process. I won't give up if things are a bit hard or challenging—I like to push myself and you soon know if what you are doing works for you.

I used to think that life happened in the future; I raced forward, always planning ahead and never truly being present in the moment. Get-up-and-go is easy for me but slowing myself down has been more challenging—and not just physically. It has been just as important for me to become aware of my mind and inner self. Yoga has really helped me achieve this balance. I started practicing yoga to become fitter, but now I use it to slow myself down and be present in the moment. Mindfulness and meditation courses have also helped to ground me. I love reading books that bring me back to the present and help me live my life more in the moment. It's a constant process of learning and growing.

Love Holly xxx

MINDSET

I now know what has enabled me to become healthy, both physically and mentally, emotionally balanced, stress-free, and content. In summary it is about:

- **Being active**
- **Enjoying a daily variety of fresh vegetables**
- **Limiting my intake of sugar, wheat, and alcohol**
- **Avoiding processed foods and always reading food labels**
- **Having "me" time**
- **Not taking life too seriously and having fun**
- **Trying new things to keep me sharp, excited, and inspired**
- **Being with positive, like-minded people who nurture a zest for life**

You do have a choice. You can learn about which are the best foods for your health and for weight loss—Amber's delicious recipes will get you on track. You can also find exercise that you enjoy and see how you can become strong, lean, and toned. Don't underestimate the importance of having time for yourself, time to rest, relax, and just be.

Every one of us can wake up in the morning and say that today, right now, this second, I am in control and I love the way I am. Are you ready?

CHANGING HABITS

It's great to embark on a healthy lifestyle and a new fitness regime feeling excited and inspired. But it's so easy to want it all to happen instantly, the old "I want it now" syndrome, so you bust a gut and cram in exercise every day. By the end of the first week you are aching but still feel positive; by the end of the second week you scream "It's taking over my life! I hate exercise!" and throw in the towel. If you haven't exercised before, or been able to maintain exercise over a long period of time, then going at it hard won't be sustainable. It's far better to ease into it slowly and build up gradually, until exercising eventually becomes part of your weekly routine. It won't happen overnight.

It's time to ditch some bad habits, too. How often when you look in the mirror do you immediately focus on what you don't like about your body? If you have negative thoughts about parts of yourself, they are often what your eyes are drawn to first: my thighs are too big, my arms are flabby, I hate the shape of my butt. Change the habit and be positive about yourself. Whenever you look in the mirror, make a point of focusing on a positive feature and pay yourself at least one compliment. Highlight your natural gifts, talent, and abilities, and don't just rate yourself in terms of appearance.

Changing habits and creating a motivational mindset is like exercising a muscle—the more you work it, the stronger it becomes. Some of our behaviors and thoughts have been with us all of our lives, so it takes time. Little things like associating the word "treat" with food (quite likely greasy, fatty, sugary food). Most of us have the connection from when we were children and our mothers would give us sweets as a reward if we behaved ourselves. There are other ways to be rewarded: treat yourself to a walk in the park or indulge in reading a good book.

EXERCISING EVENTUALLY
BECOMES PART OF YOUR
WEEKLY ROUTINE, BUT IT
WON'T HAPPEN OVERNIGHT.

TAKE THE
PRESSURE OFF

Taking the pressure off yourself is so important. If you are told not to do something, you kind of want to do it (watch your kids, they're expert at this). As soon as you restrict your diet, all you want to do is eat. And when you tell yourself you HAVE to workout, you feel pressured and try to talk yourself out of it. There is no pressure. There is no stress. If you only do half a workout then please congratulate yourself, that's great! Likewise, if you manage a brisk walk around the park, amazing—it's all about moving and getting your body active. Yes, becoming fitter, stronger, or leaner can seem like a long journey, but don't feel like you have to go at it for hours and hours—break it up into 20-minute blasts, start off small, and build up when your fitness improves. Exercising without stress or pressure makes it a choice and enjoyable.

Some training programs put you under pressure even before you begin with dubious promises: Get a dancer's body by doing this workout. Hmmm, really? These workouts can be great fun, but since the girl who is posing for the workout shots has been a dancer for the last 15 years, of course she has a dancer's body and, when you don't get a body like hers, you think you have failed. Not only is it unrealistic, frankly most of us don't have the genetic makeup to have that dancer's physique. Have your own personal goals laid out. You want to be fit and healthy for you, because that's what makes you feel good and gives you a huge sense of achievement.

Every time you work out or go to a yoga class will be different, because you are different each day. You may not have slept well; you might be more stressed or dehydrated. Don't get angry if today is harder or isn't the same as the last time you trained. Do the best you can do today; don't focus on what you did yesterday or last week but on what you are doing right now. Because your best effort today is good enough.

CHANGING THE VOICE
IN YOUR HEAD

We can make things into huge obstacles and we love to have a conversation with the voice in our head about it. You know the one that tells you it is okay to have a second cookie, but then makes you feel guilty afterward? It's a continuous battle we have with ourselves about most things.

The voice

"I've had such a stressful day at work, I need a glass of wine tonight. I know I said I wasn't going to drink all week, but after the nightmare day I've had, I deserve it. Plus, I didn't drink last night, so that's pretty good, so I can probably have a couple."

"I'm so tired I can't be bothered to go to the gym today. But I didn't go yesterday and I promised myself I would go today, so I'm going! Oh, but it's pouring with rain outside, it must be a sign to stay at home. I will go tomorrow."

WHATEVER THE MIND CAN
CONCEIVE AND BELIEVE,
IT CAN ACHIEVE.

NAPOLEON HILL.

To create a healthier lifestyle, not only do we need to change the food we eat and become more active and less stressed, but we also need to change the voice in our head to help us get there. Next time you hear the voice, don't let it talk you out of doing something positive. Try and change it to encourage and motivate you: "I can make time," "I feel so energized after a workout," "It's a bit cold outside today, but I will soon warm up."

Finding what excites you will really help to keep the voices at bay. Discover which exercises or activities you're naturally good at and do them—swimming, jogging with friends, jogging on your own, dancing, yoga, a martial art or exercise class, Pilates, or playing soccer with your kids. Keep trying new things until you find the right ones, and accept you may need to find a great teacher who inspires you or the perfect class that fits into your schedule.

We all have days when it's harder to motivate ourselves, but those sessions can turn out to be more rewarding because you know you have made the extra effort. I still have days when my little voice rears its ugly head and I don't feel like going for a run. So I have a chat with myself (now I sound slightly crazy) to remind myself how good it makes me feel, the huge sense of achievement I get afterward, the fresh air on my face, the freedom it gives me. The positives always outweigh the negatives. I change the voice from "Don't bother today, you deserve a rest" to "If I only run for 10 minutes today then that's great" and as soon as my feet hit the pavement, I know I've made the right choice and usually that 10 minutes turns into an hour.

POSITIVE
THOUGHTS

In the words of Buddha, "we are what we think." Having a positive outlook on life brings many health benefits, from reducing stress to enhancing relationships. Positive thinking has an impact on overall well-being. In our daily lives we can encounter negativity—fear, worry, dispute, jealousy, gossip, judgment—and too often it's easy to get caught up in it and then negative thoughts become a habit. Instead, try to see the glass as half full. Set your goal and visualize yourself achieving it, be it running that race or fitting into that little black dress. Having a positive attitude about exercise will boost your motivation and help you achieve your goals more easily.

Avoid negative thoughts
Don't put yourself down. Work on making your mind and body strong. Remember, it's you inside who says you can't do something, so challenge those negative thoughts and turn them into positives. Read inspiring, uplifting quotes. Find one that touches you and make it your mantra.

Be in the present
Focus your thoughts on the right now and be mindful of what is going on around you.

Be thankful
Focus every night on the things for which you are grateful and highlight all the good things in your life.

Learn to say no
By not over-committing to things, you're less likely to let people down or feel you have failed.

Surround yourself with other positive people
They will support and energize you. Being positive is contagious, in the same way as being negative is, and I know which people I'd choose to be around.

Smile
It's simple but it works.

IF IT'S IMPORTANT TO YOU, YOU WILL FIND A WAY. IF NOT, YOU WILL FIND AN EXCUSE.

NO EXCUSES!

There are many excuses that crop up when it comes to exercising, but there are always solutions, too. Do you recognize any of these excuses?

"I don't have enough time"
Even if it's a 10-minute blast, we all can find time in our day for that—every minute helps. That's 70 minutes a week, 3,640 minutes a year. And that's a lot of extra calories burned as well as a lot of endorphins—the happy hormones—released! Remember this is YOUR health and happiness you're investing in.

"I can't afford it"
You don't have to be a member of an expensive gym or invest in top-of-the-range gym equipment. All you need is your body (Okay, a pair of sneakers and a sports bra would be great, too).

"I'm not fit enough"
That's in your head; you are fit enough. Everyone began somewhere. Start at a level that works for you and build on it.

"It's too hard"
Begin with some gentle exercise and, as your fitness improves, so too will your confidence and your ability to push yourself harder.

"I don't enjoy it"
Maybe you are doing the wrong activity: it's time to try something new.

"No clean gym clothes"
Always be prepared. Double up on your gear so you always have one clean set; get it ready the night before so you're not rushing around in the morning.

"I have a baby so I can't make it to the gym"
Home workouts and DVDs are a great way to get back into shape post-baby. If that's not for you, then you can power walk/jog pushing the stroller through the park. Find another mom who also wants to get back into shape and do babysitting swaps.

"I'm just too tired"
Exercise is proven to increase your energy levels. Change the thought of "I'm too tired" into "this is really going to energize and refresh me."

"I'm injured★/I'm sick"
Okay, if it's serious maybe your body needs a rest: listen to what it's telling you. Perhaps focus on something to help prevent further injury; it might be the perfect opportunity to try something new.

★If you have an injury, ache, or pain, don't push through the pain—see a doctor. Your body and health come first; make it a priority to get a proper diagnosis, not an excuse to keep you from working out.

OBSTACLES

jump them all

Don't just focus on the things you are good at (we all have our favorite moves). Working on your weaker areas will help give you a strong and toned body. So when you see the exercise "Burpee" (page 236) in front of you (most people's least favorite move) say, "Yeah baby, bring it on!!" Keep pushing your body; it's easy to sit back into a comfort zone. You will be surprised how much your body is capable of and how quickly you will improve. Your workouts should never be easy. In fact, when they start to feel easier, it's time to make your workout more challenging. You can do this in many ways, by adding more weight, more time, or more reps. Feel the burn and fall in love with it.

Enter a race

Nothing is more motivating than having an event on the horizon, and skipping sessions becomes a lot less tempting when you've got a date set on the calendar. Raise money for your favorite charity as well. That way, everyone's a winner!

Reward yourself

When you've stuck to your training plan or reached a goal, congratulate yourself. Treat yourself to a new gym outfit, a massage, or make time for that really relaxing candle-lit bubble bath.

Visualize achieving your goal

Feel all the emotions associated with the achievement. Really focus on the details to make this experience as real as possible.

Make a date with yourself

Commit to your weekly workouts by scheduling them in your calendar. They are just as important as any meeting.

Train with a friend

Planning to do a workout with a friend is great motivation—you are less likely to skip a workout and let down your friend, and you can also spur each other on. Send a text to congratulate each other on the work you have done.

Prepare playlists that motivate you

If music be the food of love then... work out!! (Isn't that what Shakespeare said?) It's proven that a pumping beat makes you work harder, so find something that makes you want to get up and go!

Buy a nice gym outfit

Something you feel comfortable in, and don't put off buying it until you've lost weight. Your self-confidence might be a little low already so it's not going to do it any favors by wearing an old holey pair of tracksuit bottoms and your partner's baggy T-shirt.

Do it for them

Think of someone close to you and do the workout for them. When you feel you can't go on and you are ready to give up, visualize that special person and keep on going. Run that bit further, lift that bit heavier, do one more rep. It's not just for you anymore, it's for them, too.

THERE WILL ALWAYS BE OBSTACLES AND REASONS NOT TO EXERCISE, AND THAT'S WHY YOU SHOULD ALWAYS HAVE A PLAN B, OR EVEN A PLAN C, IN PLACE.

BODY

Exercise speeds up your metabolism by creating more muscle and, of course, the more intense your workout, the more calories you burn. But that does not mean exercise makes you hungrier. While a lot depends on what gender we are and our overall body composition, often we think since we've smashed our workout, we can reward ourselves with food. Mostly that's just bad habits, or your brain thinking it deserves a reward for working so hard. Studies have actually shown that the more you work out, the more you produce both appetite-suppressing proteins and hormones, so any hunger pangs might just be in your mind. Working out on an empty stomach is neither good nor bad; it's a personal choice. But what is key after exercise is making the right food choices, refueling within an hour post-workout, and making sure it's high-quality protein to repair muscle tissue. Plus, protein makes you feel fuller longer, which is an added bonus! More important than anything is to drink plenty of water to re-hydrate your body post-workout—and water also makes you feel full. So when in doubt, grab some H_2O.

EXERCISING &
THE BENEFITS

Why do we need to exercise? The bottom line is that we need to move our bodies. That's what they are designed to do. Run, jump, push, pull, bend, reach, and lift. Hundreds of years ago we didn't need to exercise—we had to be physical and active to survive. Elevators, escalators, and especially cars and computers all contribute to moving less. Our bodies are wonderful machines. To function properly, they need to be kept mobile, active, and strong.

Staying fit isn't so easy now that practically everything is done for us. Even day-to-day chores like food shopping can all be done with a click. To top it off, there's the huge choice of food we always have available at our fingertips and the added convenience of takeout, restaurants, cafés, and frozen meals. And, if we aren't preparing food ourselves, how do we really know what's in it? Not a great combo for staying fit and healthy. We need to remind ourselves why we need to be active—that it's not a chore but what our bodies require to thrive.

For many, weight loss is the main motivator to get in shape. But shifting the pounds is not just about trying to squeeze into your skinny jeans. The main reason for staying fit is to live a healthy life with greater confidence and self-esteemm and to be able to carry on with day-to-day activities such as running around with the kids, cleaning the house, carrying all the groceries, even tying our shoelaces when we are 80, feeling body-confident, living without back problems. I could go on and on...

LACK OF ACTIVITY DESTROYS THE GOOD CONDITION OF EVERY HUMAN BEING, WHILE MOVEMENT AND METHODICAL PHYSICAL EXERCISE SAVE IT AND PRESERVE IT.

PLATO

Exercise makes you feel good by releasing endorphins, the happy hormones, into your body. Just 15 minutes of exercise can improve your mood.

Exercise keeps your bones healthy—especially weight-bearing exercise, as it increases bone density, which counteracts osteoporosis.

Regular aerobic exercise lowers your blood pressure, which in turn reduces your risk of developing heart disease. Get the blood pumping and the heart racing!

Exercise speeds up your metabolism by creating more muscle. It burns body fat and calories, which will help maintain healthy weight loss. The more intense the workout, the more calories you burn. So get to it!

Exercise improves your sex life—fitter people have better sex.

Exercise gives you energy. Being active or hitting the gym is invigorating—it's the best medicine for when you're feeling sluggish.

Exercise results in smoother, more radiant, younger-looking skin because it helps pump more blood all over your body, delivering reparative nutrients to your skin's surface. It also increases collagen production making your skin appear more youthful. Yes please!

Exercise reduces stress, tension, anxiety, and boredom. It lowers the levels of cortisol, the stress hormone, in the body. Ever tried boxing? It's a super stress release.

Exercise increases the amount of blood and oxygen pumped to your brain, keeping it sharp and more

focused. Regular exercise can reduce the risk of dementia. Next time you feel mentally exhausted, try a few Jumping Jacks to reboot your brain.

Exercise strengthens and stimulates the heart and lungs, making them work more efficiently. So you can run for the bus without becoming breathless and in the long-term you could prevent the onset of heart and lung disease.

Exercise keeps your muscles strong and your body flexible. Moving your joints regularly and keeping your muscles toned will help you continue with day-to-day activities as you get older. What you put in now will be rewarded later.

Exercise improves digestion. It helps the intestinal muscles break down food. It keeps you regular (that's the nicest way of putting it).

Regular exercise helps to prevent back pain by increasing your strength, endurance, and improving your flexibility and posture. It makes you aware of the way you sit, stand, and move. Exercise keeps you more in tune with your body.

You may have heard people talking about a runner's high. Let's change that saying to an "exercise high." I can promise you it does exist and it's pretty addictive. The first few workouts may be tough: you might feel sore, out of shape, and tired, but suddenly you feel the rush—you feel strong, alive, your heart's pumping, and you feel a massive sense of achievement. When you commit to exercise, your body responds quickly and you will see huge changes in your overall body shape, your sense of well-being and confidence, and your fitness in a short span of time. Chase the buzz and feel the high.

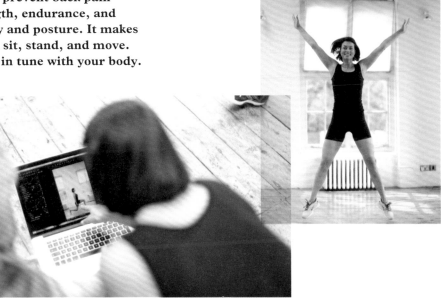

BREATHING *while* EXERCISING

Breath is life. But we take breathing for granted since we do it every second of every day without thinking about it. It's an automatic response. Breathing is the only way our blood and organs are supplied with vital oxygen. It's also one of the ways our bodies eliminate toxins and waste products. Ensuring you breathe correctly when you exercise will improve your workouts to no end. When you think about it, each breath provides your muscles with fresh oxygen. Sometimes we focus so much on what we are doing that we tend to hold our breath, and that means our muscles are denied oxygen and everything becomes so much harder. Try to learn how to breathe for these various workouts:

Strength training
During weight or resistance training, make sure you breathe out (exhale) on the effort, which is the hardest part of the exercise—usually when you are working against gravity—and inhale on the easier part. Don't worry if you get it the wrong way around; breathing in reverse is much better than not breathing at all! Likewise, when doing a push-up, inhale on the way down and exhale on the way up.

Cardio (aerobic) exercise
Take deep breaths through the diaphragm and avoid shallow breathing into the chest. You want to maintain as regular a breathing pattern as possible to maximize the oxygen flow. It doesn't matter whether you breathe through your nose or mouth or a combination of the two; everyone has a different preference.

Running
It's advisable to breathe through your mouth when running so that you can take in more oxygen. Try to find a rhythm for your breathing to help keep the inhale/exhale rate consistent. Inhale every two steps then exhale on the next two, or see if a 3:3 rhythm works better for you (inhale every three steps then exhale on the following three).

Stretching
Breathing properly while you stretch will help relax your body by bringing it back to a resting state. If you don't relax, it's easy to hold your breath and put stress and more tension on the body. Take long, deep breaths and inhale through your nose and exhale through your mouth. On every exhale, try to relax more and give in fully to the stretch.

THERE IS NOTHING WORSE THAN
DOING THE SAME THING WEEK
IN, WEEK OUT.

FORM, CORE
& POSTURE

Focus on the moment

Exercise offers you the perfect time to practice "mindfulness" and be present in the moment. While concentrating on your breathing, inhale and exhale to be fully present for the amazing thing you are doing for your body. Now is not the time to be thinking about your shopping list! This is the time to concentrate on the muscles you are working, the time to think about your toned butt, and how you are working your legs to make them lean and strong. And when it gets tough, remind yourself of the benefits of what you are doing. Tell yourself: I am becoming fitter, I am burning fat, and I am making my body lean and strong.

It's all about your form

What's form, you ask? Well, it's another way of saying how you pose and position your body for each exercise—engage your core, correct your body alignment, tighten your butt, straighten your back, etc. Form takes practice so you will want to prioritize developing it over the number of repetitions you do or how fast you can work out. Take it slowly at first. Learning good form will help you build more muscle and, more importantly, prevent injury. Always think about the muscles you are working and make sure that's where you are feeling it. Try exercising in front of a mirror. This will help increase your awareness of the way your body is moving and help to correct your form. Concentrate on all those fabulous muscles inside your body becoming strong, lean, and happy!

The secret to keeping good form is working your core (your middle, stomach, and back). Always keep your stomach muscles engaged and your back straight. If you feel pain in your back or joints such as your knees, chances are you are doing the exercise wrong. Check your alignment in the mirror. The only place you should feel the burn is in the muscles you are working.

Not only is your core good for your form, it's good for your health and love life, too!
Working your core will make you strong from the inside out. We all need to work our core because it keeps the spine and pelvis stable and provides crucial support. For women, it is particularly important to strengthen the PF (pelvic floor) and TVA (transverse abdominal), especially after giving birth when these muscles have been stretched.

Your PF is a hammock of muscles, ligaments, and sheet-like tissues that run from your pubic bone to the base of your spine. It supports your bladder, uterus, and bowel. If you've ever leaked a little urine when jumping rope, coughing, or sneezing, then you need to work on your PF. An additional bonus to having a strong PF is that it can increase sensitivity and make sex more satisfying.

Your TVA, the deepest of your core muscles, functions like a corset around your waist. Having a strong TVA is important as it protects the spine by distributing the stresses of bearing weight, thereby preventing injury and reducing the risk of lower back pain.

We're all super busy doing everyday stuff while we're sitting down, such as emailing, reading, driving, eating, or watching TV. This might lead you to develop slouched shoulders, a hunched back, or a generally bad posture. Rather than simply accepting this as a consequence of modern-day life, see it as an opportunity to develop your core as the foundation for strength. Your core is essential for balance and coordination. Core strength also helps you stay mentally strong, and when you are feeling strong and capable, life's obstacles seem a lot easier to tackle.

Sitting up straight is one of the simplest but most effective ways to improve your core strength. The act of sitting up straight immediately engages your core muscles. You grow taller, your stomach is drawn in and instantly flattens, your shoulders are gently pulled back and down. To maintain good posture you need a balance of strength and an awareness of your body—something you may have to constantly remind yourself of until it becomes second nature. It may feel awkward, even a little uncomfortable, at first. But stick with it, your body and muscles are now engaged and working.

*Here are some tips to help you find and
practice good posture:*

Sitting

Keep your legs uncrossed and your feet flat on the
floor. Your weight should be distributed evenly
between your feet, thighs, hips, and lower back.

If you can, adjust your chair so your hips are slightly
higher than your knees.

Draw your navel in toward your spine; your abs
should be firm but not too tight.

Keep your shoulders open, relaxed, and drawing down
your spine.

Make sure your ears are over your shoulders and don't
allow your chin to push forward.

Never sit for too long. Always take a break and walk
around, which helps to prevent your hamstrings and
lower back from tightening up, which can pull your
spine out of alignment.

Try sitting on an exercise ball rather than a chair while
you work.

Standing

Stand with your feet slightly apart and gently rock
back and forth so you feel the weight of your body
moving from your heels to your toes. Stop when you
feel the weight is evenly distributed over both feet.

Soften your knees and gently draw your navel in
toward your spine, keeping it firm but not too tight.

Keep your shoulders open, relaxed, and drawing down
your spine.

Make sure your ears are over your shoulders.

Imagine a line running from your earlobe through
your shoulder, hip, knee, and ankle.

In a nutshell

Back straight, shoulders squared, chin level, chest out,
stomach in! Try making these small simple corrections
to the way you sit and stand and see how your body
changes. You'll feel taller, your stomach will look flatter,
and your boobs will seem bigger. Okay, so that's on the
vanity side, but there are other reasons for developing
good posture:

To help an aching back, neck, hips, or knees.

To prevent injury when exercising.

To slow down or prevent the development of arthritis
and osteoporosis.

To boost confidence, self-esteem, and provide a sense
of empowerment.

TO MAINTAIN GOOD POSTURE,
YOU NEED A BALANCE OF
STRENGTH AND AN AWARENESS
OF YOUR BODY.

MEASURE ME UP, BABY

It's a great idea to have weekly challenges to push you out of your comfort zone. Do something you haven't done before: run further, skip longer, lift heavier weights, hold the plank position for your longest time yet, and when you feel you've reached your limits, go that little bit further.

Set yourself goals. You need to have a clear idea of what you want to achieve from your exercise routine, and map it out. Think about what you would like to achieve in a year's time and then break this down into smaller targets to reach over the coming months. Writing down your plan shows commitment and it helps to make your goals real.

Not all of your goals have to be exercise-related. Having daily targets is a great start and really works for me and for my clients. Pick five things you would like to improve or change for the next week and write them on the action plan. Give yourself a realistic target for how many times that week you are going to achieve your chosen goal. Each day give yourself a check when you've done it. Examples to try for one week might look like:

GOAL	TARGET
Drink more water	48 ounces every day
Exercise regularly	3 times a week for 45 minutes each
Avoid alcohol	5 days this week
Get more sleep	Sleep for at least 7 hours every night
Vary my cooking	Try three new healthy recipes

Fuel your body

It is best to eat within an hour of exercising. Your metabolism is fired up and your body wants some protein and nutritious food to feed your hungry muscles and speed recovery. The hour after exercise is going to be the most beneficial. If you know it's going to be hard to prepare something in that time, then make sure you have a healthy snack on hand. Eat something high in protein to aid in muscle repair: eggs, fish, seeds, and nuts are all great sources.

Your body is a furnace

When you exercise for short bursts at a higher intensity, you create the afterburn effect, which causes your body to burn more calories long after you have stopped exercising. Don't make your workout a punishment for eating badly. Eating a package of cookies because you are going to the gym later to "burn it off" isn't a healthy way to think. Being active and moving your body is an amazing gift of health you give to yourself, and exercise is the reward.

Motivate yourself

Too often we get stuck on losing weight, but jumping on the scales every day to see whether the numbers are changing can be a massively disheartening experience, especially if you don't see those numbers going down. It's also pretty stressful and stress equals more cortisol (the stress hormone), which actually holds onto body fat. Think about fat loss, not weight loss. Focus on changing your body shape and don't get obsessed about your weight. Remember that muscle weighs the same as fat. A pound is a pound, right? But a pound of muscle is far more compact—nearly 3 times smaller than fat—so takes up much less space. So if you are 140 pounds of lean muscle, you are going to look a lot better than if you are 140 pounds of fat. It's not about numbers on the scales.

Another myth is that fat turns into muscle. Fat cells can't change into muscle cells. But what you can do is burn fat and build muscle. Body fat is a storage place for extra energy when we consume more calories than we burn. Continue to do this and your fat cells increase in size. When we "burn fat," what we are doing is shrinking our fat cells. What's good to remember is that the body burns more calories maintaining muscles than it does maintaining fat. So it's time to get strong.

The jeans test

Ditch the scales and grab two pairs of jeans or two of your favorite dresses. The first pair should be a bit snug, the ones you will only pull out when you are feeling super body confident. These will be your go-to test jeans over the first few weeks of your lifestyle change. Each week, slip them on and see how they feel. Remember, things don't happen overnight. The second pair of jeans (or dress number two) should be super tight. You know these jeans, we all have them. It's the pair you've kept for years at the back of your closet, hoping one day to hop back into them. These are your 3-month target jeans. It's good to set yourself longer targets to track against your weekly goals so you can see and appreciate the results.

Measure me up, baby

Taking measurements of your body is also a good way to really see results. Make a note of them and then hide them away. Come back to them every four weeks and record your new measurements. To keep the measurements accurate, take them on exactly the same body part each time and in the same conditions. You might find it easier to get someone to help you. Wear fitted clothes or nothing at all and use a cloth measuring tape.

Arms: Measure the thickest part of your arm (usually around the bicep).

Bust: Place the measuring tape across your nipples and take the largest measurement around your chest keeping the tape parallel to the floor.

Hips: Place the measuring tape around the widest part of your hips/butt, which is usually just above your crotch.

Waist: Place the measuring tape an inch above your belly button (the narrowest part of your waist). Take the measurement after an exhale of breath. Don't suck in your tummy.

Upper thigh: Measure around the widest part of the thigh—usually about three-quarters the way up from your knee.

CARDIO & WEIGHTS

When you exercise for short bursts at a higher intensity, you create the afterburn effect, also known as EPOC (excess post-exercise oxygen consumption). This causes your body to continue to burn a higher number of calories long after you have stopped exercising. Sounds great! So by working harder for shorter bursts of time, overall you burn more calories.

If you are training for a distance run, then obviously running for a long period of time is going to benefit your training and help you reach your goal. But if you are trying to lose weight, don't spend hours on the treadmill or cross-trainer; stop watching the numbers to see how many calories you have burned. You need to mix it up and HIIT (high intensity interval train—see page 242) it! Using the HIIT method shocks your body and ramps up your metabolism for fat loss. Push yourself out of your usual comfort zone for as little as only 3 minutes. Go faster for short bursts. For example, ride the stationary bike for 3 minutes, going as fast as you can for 30 seconds, then slowing down to catch your breath for 30 seconds, repeat until you've done the fast and slower cycles each 3 times.

You will get fitter and see great results while taking only a quarter of the time.

Doing the same cardio routine can get boring, so keep it varied and find something you enjoy—cycling, swimming, or hiking perhaps. It doesn't have to mean slogging away on a treadmill. There are so many body weight exercises that really get your heart rate up, such as jumping rope, squat thrusts, mountain climbers, and burpees.

BECOME MORE CONFIDENT. WHEN YOUR BODY IS STRONG, IT POSITIVELY AFFECTS OTHER AREAS IN YOUR LIFE.

You won't get bulky

There is fear in a lot of women that if you use heavy weights you will create a big and bulky unfeminine body. I can tell you right now this is NOT true. What is bulky is fat! Lifting weights will create a leaner, more athletic, elegant-looking body.

There is one simple reason why women can't acquire muscle mass to the same degree as men, and it's down to the hormone testosterone. Women only produce a tiny amount of this hormone; men will produce roughly 20 times more. Even taking that into account, creating muscle in men still isn't easy and takes a huge amount of hard work and dedication. So don't be scared of lifting heavy weights—this is the key to making real changes to your body shape.

Top reasons why women should lift weights

Increases your metabolism and basal metabolic rate (BMR) so your body burns more calories each day.

Reduces the chance of osteoporosis by increasing bone density.

Tones and sculpts your body and gives it definition by increasing muscle tissue.

Releases the happy hormone so your mood and energy levels increase, which in turn reduces anxiety and depression.

Keeps you young—it's the most effective anti-aging activity.

Reduces many lifestyle-related diseases and chronic illnesses.

Increases quality of life and overall well-being.

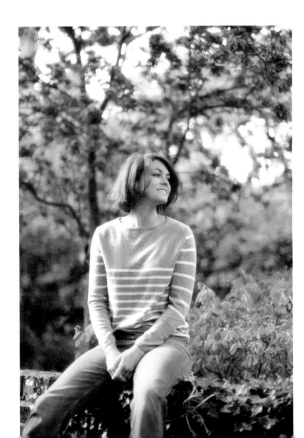

FIND THE EXERCISE YOU LOVE, WHATEVER YOUR AGE

Cardio & weight training

When you're young, your body can take the abuse of excessive late nights, binge drinking, and bad eating habits. But that doesn't mean we can't still give our bodies some TLC. Your 20s is the decade to create good lifetime habits. Now is the time to find a cardiovascular heart-pumping exercise you love, like kick-boxing, running, or cycling. When you hit your 30s, it's time to mix up your training if you haven't already. For example, if you've always been a runner, then it's time to add in weightlifting. Repeating the same thing week after week allows your body to get stuck in a "comfort zone," which means you won't be challenging your body, or your mind, but more importantly, your body will adapt to the routine and you won't increase your fitness or lose weight. You might find it harder to shift those unwanted pounds in your 30s as with each decade our metabolic base rate drops by 1 to 2 percent. If you have exercised regularly and kept a healthy lifestyle, you won't see a big difference in your body shape.

Cross training & strength training

As time goes by, you'll find shifting those extra pounds becomes harder, especially when you hit your 40s and stomach fat becomes your main enemy. Now is the time to increase your weightlifting. By lifting weights, you will preserve your lean muscle mass, which will keep your metabolic rate high so you continue to burn optimum calories. Gravity, hormones, and your slowing metabolism are a triple hit as you age, and you may find it harder to see results. But by keeping your exercise routine varied with cardio, weight, and resistance training, you will keep and can increase your muscle mass. Exercise is the answer to looking fit and feeling young. But, like it or not, as you get older, you'll have to adapt your exercise to work with your body, not against it. There is always something you can do.

Core balance & flexibility

Pilates and yoga are great ways to strengthen your core and keep your posture strong and balanced as you hit the half-century mark. And good posture is not only vital for your health, it helps you look young. Keeping your exercise up now with light weight training and moderate cardio is super important as our bones age, and lifting weights helps increase bone density, which is critical for preventing osteoporosis and breaks as you head into your 60s. Your joints and ligaments might become stiffer, so now is the time to add more stretches and also work on your balance to keep your core strength up. If you haven't tried yoga, it can be a lovely, gentle way to keep your body mobile and flexible.

No matter what your age

Young at heart and still raring to go, there are all sorts of exercises you can continue as long as you keep it varied. And continue to do the things you enjoy. There is never a cut-off point; keep active forever. It's never too late to start exercising, but take it slowly and never work through pain.

The programs I have created use functional exercises that imitate your daily activities. The aim is to make you stronger so your life gets easier and you can go about your daily tasks without risking injury. When you are not exercising, your daily routine still requires you to move—balancing, twisting, bending, pulling, and pushing are all part of everyday life, whether it's lifting your children, carrying heavy bags, or pushing the vacuum cleaner. I am not in favor of using gym machines because they make your body perform an exercise that restricts it to a certain movement, and that isn't how your body naturally moves. Learning how to do functional exercise correctly will lead to better joint mobility and general stability (a client once told me how happy she was that after exercising and learning to control her body she could now stand on the subway without having to hold on for dear life because her balance was so improved).

Variation is key to my clients' success, and that's what I have developed here; full body workouts that progress as the weeks pass but are never repeated. Your body and mind are always kept guessing and being challenged in different ways. There is nothing worse than doing the same thing week in, week out.

LET'S BEGIN

You will need:
- Gymboss app or timer.
- Jump rope: this is my favorite bit of equipment. Cheap, compact, and amazing for a cardio blast. Get a plastic or nylon one.
- Dumbbells: choose ones that weigh between 5 and 10 lbs.
- Exercise ball: this inflatable ball can double up as a chair and is great for your posture.
- A mat or even just a room with a soft carpet.

Foam roller

A bonus piece of equipment I love. You can use a foam roller to help warm up your muscles before a workout or to lengthen tight muscles post-workout. By rolling your body over the roller, you break down adhesions between the muscle fibers, allowing more blood to pump through your body. Quite like a deep tissue massage, it can be quite painful to begin with. It's great for getting those hard to reach spots like your IT band (the tendon that runs from your hip to the outside of your knee).

Tips when using the roller
- Stay on the soft tissue and don't roll over bone or joints.
- Roll over each area at least 10 times.
- If you hit a really painful spot, it's probably a trigger point. Hold for a few seconds and allow the muscle to release.

Warm Up

Any exercise program must be preceded by a warm-up and followed by a stretch (see page 208) to ensure you avoid injury. Warming up gradually increases the circulation of oxygen to your muscles, heart, and lungs, making your workout more effective. It is also a good opportunity to visualize your goals and focus on how great you will feel when you achieve them.

Complete the following movements one after the other for 20 seconds each. You're aiming to raise your heart rate as you warm up, so by the end you should feel slightly out of breath with your mind and body ready for exercise. The warm up should take 3 minutes.

CREATING YOUR OWN WORKOUT SPACE IS A GREAT IDEA. THAT WAY, IF YOU DON'T HAVE ACCESS TO A GYM OR ARE SHORT ON TIME, YOU ARE ALWAYS PREPARED FOR A HOME WORKOUT SESSION.

09

01 **March**
Bring your knees to your chest in a marching action.

02 **Down and up**
Crouch down and touch the floor, heels raised, then stand up onto your tiptoes and reach for the ceiling.

03 **Lunge with side step**
Start in a standing position and bend into a side lunge, step back to standing, and then repeat on the other side.

04 **Butt kicks**
Hopping from one leg to the other, bring your heel up to your butt.

05 **Jumping twist**
Jump while rotating your upper and lower body in different directions.

06 **Shoulder windmills**
With straight arms, rotate them both backward in big circles; repeat in a forward rotation.

07 **Fast jog and punch**
Jog in place doing a fast forward punching action.

08 **Caterpillar**
From a standing position, place both hands on the floor and walk them forward to a plank, walk them back, and return to a standing position.

09 **Downward and Upward Facing Dog**
Move in a flowing motion from one position to the next.

01

Stretch

Just as you need to warm up at the start of each workout, you should also stretch at the end. Taking the time to stretch is one of the most important parts of a workout. It provides the opportunity to relax the mind as well as the body. Picturing the muscle you are stretching and breathing "into that area" will help to relax and relieve it further.

Stretching also helps to lengthen and open your body, releasing any tension in the muscles after exercise.

Hold each stretch for 20 seconds, just at the point where it begins to feel uncomfortable. Use your breathing to relax into the stretch, inhaling and exhaling deeply. This series of stretches should take 4–5 minutes.

01 **Triceps stretch** – straighten one arm up toward the ceiling, then bend it at the elbow, taking your hand down the center of your spine. With the other hand, gently pull the elbow behind your head. To increase the stretch, interlace your fingers. Repeat on the other side.

02 **Chest and shoulder opener** – interlace your hands behind your back. Lift your straight arms away from your back. If you can, squeeze the palms of your hands together.

03 **Cat and Cow** – to stretch and open your spine. Start on all fours and slowly move from photo 03a to 03b; move fluidly for 20 seconds.

04 **Downward Facing Dog** – a wonderful full-body stretch, especially good for your hamstrings. Press your heels toward the floor and then alternate heel press.

05 **Pigeon Pose** – start on all fours, bring your right knee to your right wrist, straighten your back leg, and lower

yourself down so your right ankle is below your left hip. To increase the stretch, lower your head to the floor. Repeat on the other side.

06 **Seated spinal twist** – sit on the floor with your knees bent and slide your right foot under your left leg, placing your right foot by your left hip. Step your left foot over the right leg and place it by your right knee. Twist toward your bent knee. Repeat on the other side.

07 **Hip flexor stretch** – with your left knee pressing slightly into the floor, tuck your tailbone under and gently push your hip forward. Be careful not to sink down too deeply. To increase the stretch, raise your left arm and bend gently to the right. Repeat on the other side.

08 **Quad stretch** – from your hip flexor stretch position, reach back and pick up your back ankle, bringing your foot toward your butt. Repeat on the other side.

0 2

0 3 a

0 3 b

0 4

0 5 a

0 5 c

0 5 b

0 6

0 7

0 8

IDEALLY, LEAVE A DAY
BETWEEN EACH WORKOUT SO
YOUR BODY HAS TIME TO
RECOVER.

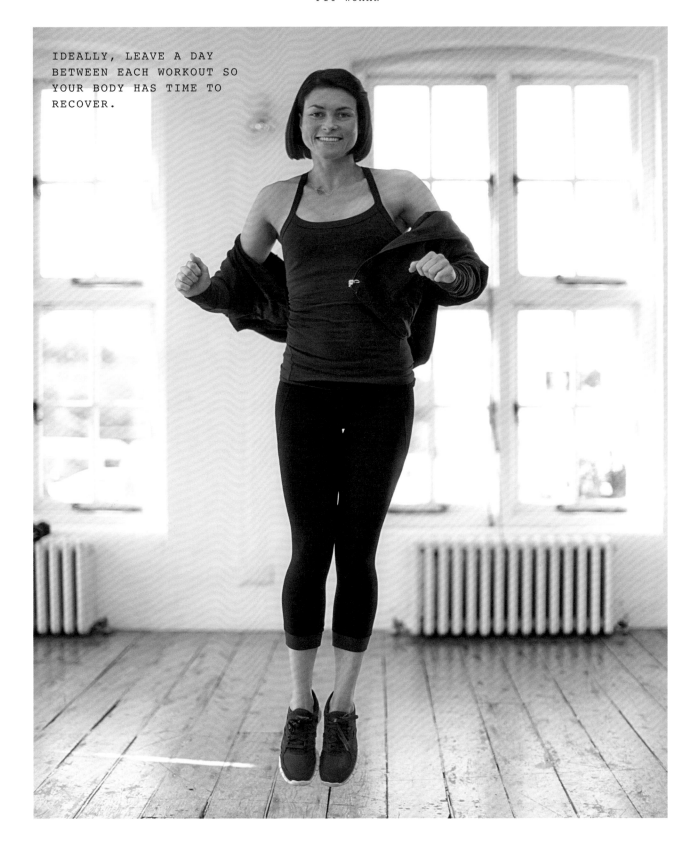

WEEK ONE

get moving

Timing
30 seconds on each exercise
15 seconds between exercises
Repeat circuit 3 times
90 seconds rest between each circuit

Tips for the week ahead

Workout 1
Make sure you get ready for the week—plan your workouts early and know which days you're exercising. Have a plan B in place just in case.

Get a good sports bra. Protect your breasts, ladies. Seriously, bouncing up and down can be not only painful but also it can stretch the tissue around your bust. Chest exercises will lift your breasts, so don't undo all that good work.

Jumping rope: don't put too much pressure on yourself to get it right the first time. Just give it a try and see what happens! If it's driving you crazy and you can't get it, then drop the rope and continue to jump with an imaginary rope.

Cardio is any form of exercise that increases your heart rate.

If you're finding things tough don't worry, we all had to start somewhere and it gets easier, I promise you! Complete the workout at your own pace, and congratulate yourself for however much you achieve today.

Workout 2
Squats are one of the best all-around exercises targeting the biggest muscles—your butt and thighs—plus they activate your core and pretty much every other muscle in your lower body. Serious fat burn. Learn to love your squats.

Feeling a bit achy today? That's normal—it just means that you worked hard. Drink plenty of water and follow the stretches at the end of each workout. It's a great time to have a magnesium bath—this essential mineral will go straight to help your aching muscles recover quickly.

Healthy snacks for the handbag: Amber's Coconut & Apricot Bliss Balls (page 91), almonds, whole-grain crackers, or apples. Don't eat them all at once though!

Today's motto: I don't FIND the time to exercise, I MAKE the time to exercise—try saying it out loud.

Workout 3
Brace your core and engage your stomach muscles. Imagine you are about to be punched in the stomach (not a very nice thought but it works!). Be sure to keep them tight throughout the whole exercise—and remember to breathe!

Remember this is a lifestyle change, so start replacing bad habits with good ones.

Mini challenge—did you know that lean muscle is 80 percent water? If you become dehydrated, your muscles won't contract properly. Give yourself the H_2O challenge today and drink at least 32 ounces of water. Try adding cucumber or lemon for that extra freshness.

How do I lift my pelvic floor? Imagine your pelvic floor is the slider of a zipper being zipped up as you lift your butt. Squeeze from the back (inside your butt) to your navel. Using visualizations like this can really help.

Week One

WORKOUT 1

3–5 minute warm-up

01 **Alternating lunge**
Thighs, butt, core
- Stand with your feet hip-width apart, hands on hips.
- Take a big step forward bending both knees; your front knee should not extend beyond your toes.
- As your back knee almost touches the floor, push back to the start and alternate legs.
- Engage your core to keep your balance throughout this move.

02 **Dips with bent knees**
Triceps, core, "chicken wings"
- Come to the edge of a chair, fingers facing forward.
- With your knees bent, lower your body, bending your elbows to 90 degrees and push back up.
- Keep your back close to the chair throughout.

03 **Jogging in place with arms raised**
Cardio, fat burn
- Raise both arms above your head.
- Jog in place, bringing your knees up as high as you can and lifting your feet off the ground.

04 **Plié squat**
Inner thigh, butt, core
- Stand with your feet wider than shoulder-width apart—toes pointing out (second position for any ballerinas out there).
- With your back straight, lower your body so your knees are in line with your toes.
- Push through your heels back up to starting position.
- Remember to keep your shoulders back, engaging your core, abs, and pelvic floor.

05 **Kneeling press-up**
Chest, shoulders, triceps, core
- Get on all fours.
- Walk your hands forward one hand space.
- Shift your weight forward so your shoulders are over your hands.
- Bend your arms with your elbows pointing backward and lower your body.
- As your chest almost touches the floor, push up back to the starting position.
- Keep your head in line with your body throughout.

06 **Jump rope**
Cardio, fat burn
- Hold the jump rope handles at hip level with the rope on the floor behind you.
- Flick your wrists and swing the rope over your head.
- Just before it hits the floor jump, keeping both feet together.

To finish
4-minute stretch

Week One

WORKOUT 2

3–5 minute warm-up

01 **Side lunge**
Inner thigh, outer thigh, butt, core
- Stand tall with your back nice and straight.
- Take a big step to one side.
- Bend your landing leg to 90 degrees.
- Push your hips back, keeping your bent knee over your ankle.
- With a big push, come back up to standing and repeat on the other side.

02 **Arm curl to shoulder press**
Biceps, shoulders, core
- Stand with your feet hip-width apart and with a slight soft bend in the knees.
- Hold the weights at your sides and engage your core.
- With your palms facing upward, curl the weights up to your shoulders.
- Open your arms out so your palms now face forward.
- Press the weights from your shoulders to above your head.
- Slowly reverse the move back through the curl.

03 **Squats**
Thighs, butt, core
- Stand tall with your feet shoulder-width apart. You can place an exercise ball behind you, if you wish (as shown).
- Hold your arms straight out in front of you at shoulder height.
- Keep your back straight and bend your knees until your butt just touches the ball.
- Push your hips back and keep your weight over your heels.
- Stand back up and repeat.

04 **Crouch Jumping Jacks**
Cardio, fat burn

- Start with your feet together, crouch down, and bend at the knees so your fingers can touch the floor.
- Jump up and spread out your arms and legs to form an X shape.
- Jump straight back down into your crouch position and repeat.

05 **Back raise**
Upper back, shoulders

- Lie down on your front.
- Spread out your arms so you are making a T shape, palms facing down.
- With your thumbs up, raise your arms and upper body off the floor; arching your upper back slightly.
- Pause and slowly lower yourself back down to the starting position.
- Don't press your stomach into the ground; use your back muscles to raise up.

06 **Egg Roll**
Abs, core, balance

- Sit upright on the floor.
- Bring your knees toward your body, keeping your feet together and flat on the floor.
- Keeping your hands on your shins, round your back and tuck your tailbone under.
- Roll back onto your shoulders in a nice smooth action, ensuring that you do NOT roll back onto your neck, then roll back to the starting position.

To finish
4-minute stretch

Week One

WORKOUT 3

3–5 minute warm-up

01 Backward lunge
Thighs, butt, calves, core
- Stand with your feet hip-width apart, with your hands on your hips.
- Take a big step backward, bending both knees to 90 degrees with the back knee almost touching the floor. Remember to engage your core.
- Push back to the start and repeat, alternating your legs.

02 Plank with pelvic floor squeeze
Core, arms
- Get on all fours with your hands under your shoulders.
- Straighten your legs, pushing your heels back.
- You should now be in a nice straight line from head to ankles.
- Brace your core, keeping your body firm, and squeeze your pelvic floor (see tip on page 211).

03 Flies on the floor
Chest, core
- Lie on your back with your knees bent and your feet hip-width apart.
- Grab a weight in each hand and hold them above you in line with your shoulders, palms facing each other.
- Engage your core and slightly bend your arms.
- Lower your arms to an inch away from touching the floor. Pause and return to the start position.

04 **Hips raised bridge with pelvic floor squeezes**
Back, butt, thighs, core
- Lie on your back with your knees bent and your feet hip-width apart.
- Engage your stomach muscles and zip up your pelvic floor.
- Push your heels into the floor to raise your hips.
- Your body should be in a straight line from your shoulders to your knees.
- Hold this position and squeeze and release your pelvic floor.

05 **Single dumbbell pullover**
Back, arms, core
- Lie on your back with your knees bent and your feet hip-width apart.
- Hold one weight straight above you with both hands and engage your stomach muscles.
- With a slight bend in your elbows, lower the weight back over your head toward the floor.
- When the weight is an inch or so from the floor, pause and lift back to the start position.

06 **Jump rope**
Cardio, fat burn
- Hold the jump rope handles at hip level with the rope on the floor behind you.
- Flick your wrists and swing the rope over your head.
- Just before it hits the floor, jump, keeping both feet together.

To finish
4-minute stretch

WEEK TWO

get strong

Timing
40 seconds on each exercise
15 seconds between exercises
Repeat circuit 3 times
90 seconds rest between each circuit

Tips for the week ahead

Workout 1

Be proud of the changes you are making, no matter how small, and don't forget the value of a workout. It's about how it makes you feel, not just how many calories you burn.

Cardio HIIT! Give it everything you have. Getting your heart rate up for short bursts maximizes your fat-burn and is great for fitness.

Let's go nuts. Walnuts contain more antioxidants, folic acid, and vitamin E than any other nut, plus you get your essential omega-3 fats. Tasty too!

Workout 2

The SOS wave (page 222) is for balance. It's a body and mind exercise to focus on your core, coordination, and concentration. When these three are top of their game, your workouts will be accelerated.

Think of getting enough sleep as being just as important as eating a healthy diet and getting regular exercise. Getting 7 hours of sleep after a day of healthy eating and moderate exercise can lower the risk of heart disease by up to 65 percent.

Mini challenge: try getting 7 hours sleep tonight.

Workout 3

Do you have that Friday feeling? Remember, everything in moderation; don't wake up with a hangover tomorrow. You know you'll regret it.

Don't make excuses for why you can't get your exercise done. Focus on all the reasons why you must make it happen.

Halfway there, well done! Set your goals and targets for next week. Write them down or tell someone about them. Make them real and make them happen.

Week Two

WORKOUT 1

3–5 minute warm-up

**01 Backward lunge with knee raise
(20 seconds each side)**
Thighs, calves, core, butt, balance
• Stand tall with your feet hip-width apart.
• Take a big step backward, bending both knees to 90 degrees with the back knee almost touching the floor. Remember to engage your core.
• With a big push off the back foot, drive your back knee up toward your chest.
• Take the lifted leg straight back into the backward lunge position and repeat.

02 Mountain climbers
Cardio, fat burn, core, legs, shoulders
• Get into a high plank position with your shoulders above your hands and your heels pushing back.
• Keep your body in a straight line from your head to your heels—no high butts please.
• Bring one knee toward your chest and tap your toe to the floor.
• Moving quickly, repeat with the other leg and continue alternating.
• Keep your stomach muscles engaged throughout to feel the burn.

03 Triceps kick back
Triceps, core
• Grab your weights and stand with your feet hip-width apart, knees slightly bent.
• Engage your core and lean forward from the hips so your butt sticks out with your arms by your sides and elbows bent.
• Keeping your elbows close to your body, straighten your arms back behind you.
• Pause and squeeze your triceps (the muscle on the back of your arm).
• Bring your arms back to the start and repeat.

04 **Chest press with table top legs**

Chest, triceps, core

- Grab your weights in each hand and lie on your back, feet off the ground and knees in line with your hips.
- Gently press your back into the floor and engage your stomach muscles.
- Hold the weights straight above you in line with your shoulders and palms away.
- Bend your elbows and lower the weights until your arms touch the floor (elbows at 90 degrees).
- Push back up into the start position and repeat.

05 **Superman with pelvic floor squeeze (20 seconds per leg and arm)**

Butt, back, core, pelvic floor

- Get on all fours, hands under your shoulders and knees under your hips.
- Keep your back flat and your stomach muscles engaged.
- Straighten your left leg back behind you and raise it so your ankle is in line with your hip, so you have a straight line from your head to your ankle.
- Squeeze your butt as you lift your leg.
- At the same time, raise your right arm straight out in front of you.
- Return back to all fours and repeat.

06 **Modified squat thrust on exercise ball against a wall**

Cardio, fat burn, core, leg, shoulders

- Place an exercise ball against a wall and get into the plank position with your hands on the ball.
- Engage your stomach muscles, creating a strong core.
- Jump your feet in toward your chest and straight back out to the starting position and repeat.
- Keep your core engaged and your butt down throughout the interval.

To finish
4-minute stretch

Week Two

WORKOUT 2

3–5 minute warm-up

01 Walking lunge with weights
Thighs, butt, core
- Stand with your feet hip-width apart, holding your weights by your sides.
- Take a big step forward and bend both knees; your front knee shouldn't extend beyond your toe.
- As your back knee almost touches the floor, push off your back foot and take a big step forward, bending both knees.
- Keep your core engaged to help with balance and use the length of your room to walk your lunges forward.

02 Jump rope
Cardio, fat burn
- Just as we did in Week One (see page 217).
- If you feel ready, try to pick up the speed.
- Move onto a single jump.

**03 Single leg balance with SOS wave
(20 seconds per leg)**
Core, balance, upper back, shoulders
- Stand tall with your feet hip-width apart with your arms by your sides, palms facing forward.
- Find a spot at eye level to focus on.
- Engage your core and shift your weight onto your left leg.
- Bend your right leg and raise your knee to your chest as high as you can.
- Keeping good balance, slowly lift your arms away from your sides and above your head, squeezing your shoulder blades. Repeat, alternating legs.

04 Modified burpee (squat thrust with jump)
Cardio, fat burn, core, legs
- Start with your hands on a chair or a step (the higher you are, the easier you are making it) and keep your legs straight back behind you.
- Engage your core and keep your abs tight throughout.
- You should be in a straight line from head to ankles as in a high plank.
- Don't let your hips drop down.
- Jump both feet toward your chest and take the weight in your legs.
- From here, jump straight up, reaching your arms in the air.
- Once landed, return back to start position and repeat.

05 Kneeling press-ups
(as in Week One, Workout 1, but more challenging)
Chest, triceps, core
- Start in a high plank position with your hands under your shoulders.
- Bend your knees and lower to the floor.
- With your elbows facing backward, lower your body until your chest almost touches the floor.
- Pause at the bottom and push back to the start position.

06 Fast feet with sprinter's arms
Cardio, fat burn
- Stand up on the balls of your feet with your knees slightly bent and leaning slightly forward.
- Break into a fast run on the spot.
- Move your arms and feet as fast as you can.
- Imagine a 100m sprint and you are going to win it!

To finish
4-minute stretch

Week Two

WORKOUT 3

3–5 minute warm-up

01 **Dumbbell swing**
Butt, abs, core
- Stand tall with your feet shoulder-width apart, holding one weight in front of you with both hands.
- Keeping your back straight, lower into a squat, keeping your body weight in your heels and swinging your weight in front of you.
- Push into your heels and thrust your hips forward as you stand up tall.
- With straight arms, swing your weight above your head.
- Make sure your abs are tight and your core is engaged throughout.
- Swing the weight to the start position and repeat, keeping a fluid motion throughout.

02 **Plank into side arm balance**
Core, waist, shoulders
- Get into a high plank position with your feet hip-width apart.
- Keep a straight line from your head to your ankles and your hands beneath your shoulders.
- Reach up to the sky with one hand, turning your body as you do, so that you are balancing in a T shape.
- Bring your arm back to the start position on the floor and repeat on the other side.
- Keep your body straight and your core engaged throughout.

03 **Dry swimming**
Back
- Lie on your front, arms out straight ahead.
- Keeping your legs together, raise them off the floor and hold.
- Raise your chest and arms off the floor and do a breast stroke motion, looking at the floor.
- Don't push your stomach into the floor; make sure your back does the work.

04 **Plank straddle jumps**
Cardio, fat burn, core, abs, shoulders, legs
- Get into a high plank position.
- Keep a straight line from your head to your ankles and your hands beneath your shoulders.
- Keep your core tight and zip up your pelvic floor.
- Jump your legs out wide and then jump them straight back together.
- Don't cheat; keep your butt down throughout.

05 **V shaped legs**
Inner thighs, abs, core
- Lie on your back with your feet straight up in the air, feet flexed.
- Slightly press your lower back into the floor and draw your stomach in, engaging your pelvic floor and core.
- Open your legs as wide as you can, pause, and slowly bring them back to the start position. Repeat.

06 **Egg Roll**
Core, abs, balance
- Sit upright on the floor.
- Bring your knees toward your body, keeping your feet hip-width apart and flat on the floor.
- Keep your hands together on your shins, round your back, and tuck your tailbone under.
- Roll back onto your shoulders in a nice smooth action, ensuring you do not roll back onto your neck.
- Roll back to the starting position, reaching forward with your arms and trying to raise your butt off the floor. Repeat.

To finish
4-minute stretch

WEEK THREE

get lean

***

Timing
50 seconds on each exercise
10 seconds between exercises
Repeat circuit 3 times
60 seconds rest between each circuit

Tips for the week ahead

Workout 1
Spending time exercising and strengthening your back is a surefire way to have a happy, healthy, pain-free back.

Don't ever skip breakfast. It will fire up your metabolism for the day and keep you from grabbing a sugary, fatty snack later on.

Don't think lifting weights is going to bulk you up; think lean and strong. After a workout with weights your metabolism is raised for hours after— meaning you'll still be burning fat while you are sitting at your desk!

Workout 2
Make sure you have rest days, because these are times for your muscles to repair and heal. Days off are just as important as days on.

High protein meals are what you should have after a workout. Protein goes straight to repair your tissues and it's what your body is crying out for. Try Quinoa with a Rainbow of Jewels (page 62) or Baked Haddock (page 76).

When it comes to the Egg Roll, don't worry if you spend more time on your butt than on your feet. Keep trying and don't forget to laugh: remember exercise is fun!

Pain in your lower back? Make sure to check your form and focus on engaging your core while you exercise. You should never feel pain in your back or your knees.

Workout 3
A million abdominal crunches won't give you a flat stomach—Russian twists, squats, woodchops, planks, and keeping good posture will. And stick to your healthy eating. Bring on that flat stomach!

Bounding, jumping rope, and jumping are all great for increasing bone density.

Week Three

WORKOUT 1

3–5 minute warm-up

01 **Squat thrusts**
Cardio, fat burn, core, abs, legs, shoulders
- Assume the high plank position with your arms straight and your shoulders over your hands.
- Engage your stomach muscles creating a nice strong core.
- Jump your feet in toward your chest and straight back out to the starting position and repeat.
- Keep your core engaged throughout and your butt down.

0 1

02 **Thumbs out dorsal raise on exercise ball**
Back, shoulders, balance
- Lie down with your front on an exercise ball with your toes touching the floor.
- Spread your arms out so you are forming a T shape.
- With your thumbs up, raise your arms and upper body off the ball, keeping your toes on the floor and hips on the ball.
- Pause and slowly lower back to the starting position.

0 2

03 **Weighted lunge with bicep curl**
Thighs, butt, biceps, core
- Grab your weights and stand with your feet hip-width apart.
- Hold the weights by your side with your palms facing forward.
- Take a big step forward bending both knees; your front knee should not go beyond your toes.
- As your back knee almost touches the floor, hold the position and curl the weights up toward your shoulders.
- Push back to the start, lowering the weights.
- Repeat, alternating legs.

0 3

04 **Weighted squat to shoulder press**
Thighs, butt, core, shoulders
- Grab your weights and stand tall with your feet shoulder-width apart.
- Hold your weights at shoulder height with a bent elbow.
- Keep your back straight and bend your knees until your knees are at 90 degrees.
- Push your hips back and keep your weight over your heels.
- Stand back up, lifting the weights above your head as you reach standing position.
- Lower the weights back to shoulder level and repeat.

05 **Knee to chest and donkey kick (25 seconds each side)**
Balance, butt, core
- Stand tall with your feet hip-width apart, arms by your side.
- Bring one knee up toward your chest.
- Keeping a straight back, bending from the hip, and keeping your arms still, kick your raised leg back behind you, allowing your body to come forward.
- Return to standing position and repeat with the other leg.

06 **Side plank (25 seconds each side)**
Cardio blast, fat burn, core, leg, shoulders
- Lie on your side.
- Place your elbow directly beneath your shoulder.
- Raise your hips off the ground and reach to the ceiling with your left arm so your body is in a straight line from head to heels.
- After 25 seconds, gently lower, turn over, and repeat on the other side.

To finish
4-minute stretch

Week Three

WORKOUT 2

3–5 minute warm-up

01 Elevated back lunge (25 seconds per side)
Thighs, butt, core, balance
• Stand tall in front of a chair or step, take a big step forward, and place your back foot on the chair or step.
• Bend your front knee and lower your body without leaning forward, keeping your back straight.

01

02 Suitcase swing
Butt, legs, core
• Grab your weights and stand tall with your feet hip-width apart.
• Imagine that your weights are suitcase handles.
• Lower into a squat, keeping your body weight in your heels and swinging your weights behind you.
• Push into your heels as you stand up tall.
• With straight arms, swing your weights above your head.
• Make sure your abs are tight and your core is engaged throughout.

02

03 Full press-up and kneeling press-up
Chest, triceps, core, abs
• Assume the plank position.
• Gently lower your body toward the floor keeping your elbows pointing backward.
• Keep your core engaged and your stomach tight—your body should be in a straight line from head to heels.
• As your body almost touches the floor, push back up.
• Now come onto your knees and perform 3 kneeling push-ups as in Week Two, Workout 2.

03

04 **Crouch Jumping Jacks (as in Week One, Workout 2)**
Cardio, fat burn
- Stand tall with your feet together, heels off the floor, on your tip toes.
- Lower your butt down to your heels and place your fingertips on the floor in front of you.
- Jump up and spread your arms and legs out to make an X shape.
- Land straight back into your crouch position and repeat.

05 **Low side plank with arm raise (25 seconds each side)**
Waist, back, shoulders, core
- Lie down on your right side holding a weight in your left hand. Raise into a low side plank as we did in Week Three, Workout 1 (see page 229).
- Start with the weight at your left hip and, with a straight arm, raise it into a T position.
- Lower the weight back to your hip and repeat for 25 seconds.
- Swap sides and repeat.

06 **Egg Roll to stand (as in Week Two, Workout 3, but finishing in a standing position)**
Cardio blast, fat burn, core, leg, shoulders
- Perform the exercise as for Week Two, but as you roll forward and swing your arms forward, use the momentum to come onto your feet, pushing into your heels and standing up tall.
- Bend your knees to sit back onto the floor and repeat.
- Too hard? Use your hands to give you a little push as you begin to stand up, or stay with the Week Two version.

To finish
5-minute stretch

Week Three

WORKOUT 3

3–5 minute warm-up

01 **Jump rope (as in Week One, Workout 1)**
Cardio
• Try to pick up the pace a little with smooth
single jumps.

02 **360-degree lunge (front/side/back weighted)**
Inner, outer, front, and back thigh, core
• This move brings together the forward, side, and
back lunges we have been doing in the first couple
of weeks.
• Stand tall with your feet hip-width apart and
holding your weights by your sides.
• Perform a forward lunge and push back into
the standing position.
• With the same leg, move into a side lunge, pushing
back into the standing position.
• With the same leg, step back into a backward lunge.
• From the standing position, repeat with the other leg.

03 **Woodchop (25 seconds each side)**
Back, thighs, shoulders, core, waist
• Stand tall with your feet shoulder-width apart, holding
a single weight with both hands.
• Squat down, touching the weight on your left foot.
• Stand back up while raising the weight above your
right shoulder.
• Twist from left to right, bringing your left heel off the
ground as you reach up.
• Imagine you are chopping down a tree.
• Repeat, alternating from your right foot to your
left shoulder.

04 **Russian twists**

Waist, back, core

- Sit on the floor with your feet together, heels on the floor and knees bent.
- Hold a weight with both hands slightly in front of your body.
- Lean back a few inches (slightly) and engage your abs.
- Twist so the weight is moving from one side to another.
- Picture yourself rowing down the Amazon in a canoe.

05 **High plank on exercise ball**

Core, shoulders, abs

- Get onto all fours with an exercise ball at your feet.
- One leg at a time, place your feet and shins on the ball.
- Assume the high plank position with both feet and shins steadily on the ball.
- Be sure to engage your core and tense those abs to keep a nice straight line from your head all the way down to your heels.

06 **Low side plank (25 seconds per side)**

Waist, core

- Lie on your side.
- Place your right elbow directly beneath your shoulder.
- Raise your hips off the ground so your body is in a straight line from head to heels.
- Lift your left arm up into a T shape then lower, wrapping it under your body.
- After 25 seconds, gently lower, turn over, and repeat on the other side.

To finish

5-minute stretch

WEEK FOUR

get hooked

Timing

60 seconds on each exercise
0 seconds between exercises
Repeat circuit 3 times
30 seconds rest between each circuit

Tips for the week ahead

Workout 1

Burpees (page 236) are the king of cardio and the more burpees you do, the quicker you'll see results. Turn that hate into love and watch the fat melt off.

Your glute (butt) muscle is the biggest in your body. The more muscle you have, the more calories your body burns, even when resting. Fire up your glutes and make that muscle burn today.

As the saying goes "Fail to prepare, prepare to fail," so get your healthy food ready the night before and always have your healthy snacks on hand.

Workout 2

Triceps—banish those chicken wings! Get the biggest muscle in your arm burning for that lean and toned look.

If you still look cute at the end of your workout, then you didn't train hard enough. Sweat and red faces are all good when it comes to exercising!

When it gets tough, smile to yourself and be content. You are doing a wonderful thing for your body right now!

Any exercise where you have weights above your head is amazing for strengthening your abs.

The Crazy monkey (page 239) is a great core exercise, so make sure your core is tight and engaged throughout.

Workout 3

You should be feeling fit and strong—well done for getting this far. There's no rest in between each exercise—feel the burn and don't give up. The wonderful feeling of "I did it!" at the end of this workout will be a great reward for all your effort.

Week Four

WORKOUT 1

3–5 minute warm-up

01 **Burpee**
Cardio, fat burn, full body
- Assume the high plank position (see Week One, Workout 3).
- Engage your core and jump your knees toward your chest as in a squat thrust.
- Smoothly transfer your weight to your legs, keeping your feet beneath your knees.
- From this crouching position, jump up while reaching up with your hands.

01

02 **Bridge with single leg raise**
Butt, back, thighs, core
- Lie on your back with your knees bent and feet hip-width apart.
- Engage your stomach muscles and zip up your pelvic floor. Push your heels into the floor to raise your hips.
- Hold this position and raise one leg off the ground so your knee is above your hip.
- Return your leg to the floor and then repeat the raise with the other leg. Try to keep your hips level.

02

03 **Curtsy to knee raise with shoulder press**
(30 seconds per leg)
Butt, thighs, shoulders, balance, core
- Stand tall with your feet hip-width apart and weights by your side.
- Step back with your right foot so it goes behind and outside the line of your left foot.
- Keeping your back straight, bend both legs so your front knee is at 90 degrees and you look as if you are curtsying. Touch the weights to the floor on either side of your front foot and in line with your shoulders.
- Push back up and bring your knee to your chest.
- Raise the weights above your head.
- Repeat with the other leg.

03

04 **Jump rope**

Cardio, fat burn

- Our old favorite (see Week One, Workout 1).
  If you feel ready to step it up, start running in
  place while skipping.
- Drive those knees high as if you were sprinting.

05 **Jack-knife on exercise ball**

Abs, shoulders, balance, core

- Get into a high plank position with your feet and
  shins on an exercise ball (see Week Three, Workout 3).
- Engage your core and tense your abs to keep you
  nice and straight.
- Bring your knees up to your chest, rolling the ball
  under your shins and feet as you go.
- Keep your back straight and your shoulders
  over your hands.

06 **Flies on exercise ball**

Cardio blast, fat burn, core, leg, shoulders

- Grab your weights and sit on an exercise ball.
- Walk your feet forward until just your head and
  upper back are on the ball.
- Raise the weights up with your arms in line with
  your shoulders.
- Engage your core and legs to keep stability on the ball.
- With palms facing each other and your arms slightly
  bent, lower the weights until your elbows are in line
  with your body.
- Raise back up to the starting position and repeat. Keep
  your hips lifted throughout and feel the burn.

To finish

5-minute stretch

Week Four

WORKOUT 2

3–5 minute warm-up

01 Plié squat with high pull
Inner thighs, butt, upper back, core
- Grab your weights and stand with your feet wider than shoulder-width apart with your toes and knees pointing outward—remember second position, ballet dancers.
- Hold the weights straight down in front of you, palms facing toward you.
- Keeping your back straight, squat down, making sure your knees stay in line with your toes.
- As you stand up, raise your elbows high to bring the weights under your chin.
- Keeping your shoulders relaxed, squeeze your shoulder blades together.
- Lower your arms and sit straight back into your plié squat.

01

02 Single arm row to extension (T raise) (30 seconds per side)
Butt, back, thighs, core
- Stand tall with your feet shoulder-width apart and a weight in your right hand.
- Take a lunge to your left. Place your left arm on your left thigh for support and hold.
- Start with the weight on the floor and, keeping your arm close to your body, lift the weight.
- When your arm is in line with your body twist, extend your arm and raise the weight above you, looking up to your raised hand.
- Slowly return to the start position, repeat for 30 seconds, and switch sides.

02

03 Running in place with weights above your head
Cardio, legs, shoulders, core
- Grab your weights and hold them straight above your head. Tighten and engage your core.
- Run in place by bringing your knees up to your chest.

03

04 **Tricep dips**

Triceps, core, balance

- Sit on the edge of a chair with your hands on the chair, fingers facing forward.
- Either keep your legs straight out in front of you or rest them on an exercise ball.
- Taking your weight in your arms, lower your body toward the floor, keeping your back close to the chair.
- Bend your elbows to 90 degrees and push back up.
- Your triceps will burn, but don't forget that your core is always working.

05 **Crazy monkey (handstand leg kicks)**

Shoulders, back, abs, core, legs

- Place your hands on the floor under your shoulders.
- Bend your knees and stick your butt in the air.
- Keep your weight over your hands and jump your feet off the floor, trying to kick your butt with your heels.
- Go as high as you can—think handstand and one day you might get there—have fun!

06 **Lunge with weighted rotation**

Thighs, butt, waist, core

- Grab one weight and hold it in both hands close to your chest.
- Step forward into a lunge and, as you do this, rotate your body so it is facing over your front leg.
- Keep your back straight and core strong.
- Push back to the start position and repeat on the other side.

To finish

5-minute stretch

Week Four

WORKOUT 3

3–5 minute warm-up

01 **Jumping scissor lunges**
Cardio blast, fat burn, legs, butt
- Step forward into a lunge position, but only drop half as deep into the lunge.
- Quickly jump up and switch legs mid-air, landing softly on opposite legs.
- Keep your back straight.
- This move should be fast and dynamic.

02 **Balancing tricep kickbacks (30 seconds on each side)**
Triceps, butt, legs, core
- Grab your weights and stand with your feet hip-width apart.
- Balance on one foot and bend forward from the hips.
- Extend your raised leg behind you, letting it bend slightly.
- Keep your elbows close to your sides and straighten your arms, lifting the weights up in line with your sides. Focus on a spot in front of you to maintain your balance.

03 **Squatting wall sit**
Butt, thighs, shoulders, arms
- Get into a squat position, pressing your lower back and shoulders flat against the wall.
- Make sure your butt is in line with your knees and your thighs are parallel to the floor. Keep your knees over your ankles.
- Hold your squat and extend your arms straight out in front of you.
- Rotate your arms from the "thumbs up" position to the "thumbs down" position for a full 60 seconds.

04 **Straddle jump with kneeling press-up**
Cardio, fat burn, chest, triceps, abs
- Get into the high plank position (see Week One, Workout 1).
- Keep your core engaged and your stomach tight—your body should be in a straight line from head to heels.
- Jump your feet wide to a straddle then back to the start.
- Place your knees on the floor and do a kneeling press-up.
- Repeat in this pattern.

05 **Mountain climbers**
Cardio, fat burn, shoulders, abs, legs
- Start in the high plank position (see Week One, Workout 1).
- Bring one knee into your chest.
- Quickly swap legs and bring the other knee to your chest.
- Keep changing legs as fast as you can while maintaining the plank position.

06 **Saucer**
Abs, thighs
- Lie on your back with your arms by your sides.
- Bring your legs into a tabletop position—knees over hips and ankles in line with knees.
- Engage your core and gently press your lower back into the floor.
- Lift your head, chest, and arms off the floor. Extend your legs in front of you at 45 degrees. Hold for 60 seconds.
- If this is too much, bring your legs back into the start position and raise your arms and body only.

07 **Squat thrust**
Abs, thighs
- Start in a high plank position (see Week One, Workout 1).
- Jump your feet as close to your hands as you can.
- Then jump both feet back into a high plank. Repeat.

To finish
5-minute stretch

Don't have time?

TIME TO TABATA!

Tabata training is seriously effective at burning fat and improving cardio. It's a workout that is super short (4 minutes in total) and done with super high intensity.

This training technique was created by Izumi Tabata, a Japanese scientist, in the early 1990s after carrying out tests on two groups of athletes. The first undertook moderate intensity workouts, lasting an hour, and the second were trained to do high intensity interval training (HIIT) workouts lasting only 4 minutes: 20 seconds of all-out effort followed by a 10-second rest, repeated eight times. The results showed that HIIT increased the aerobic and basal metabolic rate of anyone who used it.

HIIT or Tabata training fires up your metabolism during the workout and keeps it fired up long after you have finished, creating the afterburn effect. So you continue to burn calories long after your workout has finished, which increases your metabolism. Having a high metabolism will help you burn fat. The benefits for this high intensity training are clear, but it should be used in addition to, not as a replacement for, other types of training. It's all about getting a balance and keeping it varied.

Tabata is for people who have successfully made it through my four-week workout program (pages 211–241). Because of its high intensity, Tabata could be dangerous for anyone at risk for strokes and heart attacks. If you have high blood pressure, consult with your doctor before performing Tabata or HIIT exercises.

Now to give it a try. First download the Tabata or Gymboss interval timer app to help you keep to your 4-minute workout. Remember it's 20 seconds of all your effort and a 10-second rest. Make sure you have warmed up properly before you start a Tabata workout.

The aim is to give it everything you have—20 seconds to kill it! You do eight rounds in total. Each exercise lasts for 20 seconds with 10 seconds rest. Do all four exercises, one after the other, then repeat. Done!

Tabata Workout 1
• 20 seconds of Burpees (page 236)
10 second rest
• 20 seconds of Mountain climbers (page 241)
10 second rest
• 20 seconds of Fast feet with sprinter's arms (page 223)
10 second rest
• 20 seconds of Press-ups (page 230)
Repeat

Tabata Workout 2
• 20 seconds of Squat thrusts (page 228)
10 second rest
• 20 seconds of Crouch jumping jacks (page 215)
10 second rest
• 20 seconds of Caterpillar walkouts (page 207)
10 second rest
• 20 seconds of Egg Rolls to stand (page 231)
Repeat

CONCLUSION

After all is said and done, after all the kids are ready for school with bags packed and out the door, after all those early starts getting to work, cold and dark in the middle of a frosty winter's morning, after all those late nights, sitting at the computer writing into the wee hours of the morning, it's easy to forget the love that we need to give to ourselves.

There is a certain love and care that we should all give ourselves daily and there are many trappings that we can fall into in modern life, but there is a way to make things easier and more enjoyable, to be able to live life with a little more joy and contentment. This book has been, for the three of us, a way of putting all the things we share with each other in one place. It's a book to remind ourselves of how to hold onto that joy and stay content—we all need to be reminded of how to do that sometimes.

In some moments, life can get a little unmanageable and we can start to slip. It's best to just draw a line through that moment and start again, without any judgment and without giving yourself a hard time.

We are all constantly looking to learn and grow, yet we still mess up and we still make mistakes. We are far from perfect, but it's important to each of us to maintain a sense of self-love and self-awareness and to continue trying our best.

On the pages of this book we don't propose a hardcore regime—it's a book that you can pull off the shelf time and time again to gain inspiration and get back on track, at any time of year.

It's been a huge privilege, lots of hard work, and endless laughs for us to write this book. We hope you have as much fun with it as we have had writing it.

With love from Sadie, Holly, and Amber xxx

KNOWLEDGE IS POWER

BE PREPARED

Relying solely on your willpower is risky, and it's not likely to work. It's better to be prepared instead. If you go too long without food, your blood sugar levels will drop and that's when you'll find yourself tempted by a quick fix—usually high sugar and trans fat snacks. You can try to avoid this by not having anything unhealthy in the house in the first place, and making sure you always carry a healthy snack with you for when you're out.

Read your labels

Get wise to packaging. You will be surprised by what's actually in so-called "natural," "healthy," "organic," "fresh," "low-fat" food products. Lots of these cleverly marketed packaged foods and snacks are not so good for you at all—so read labels carefully. Foods are often filled with stabilizers, emulsifiers, E-numbers, high-fructose sweeteners, corn syrup, and other equally nasty ingredients. "Low-fat" products are some of the worst—when taking out the fats, sugar is often added to combat the loss of flavor, which makes it even worse for you. Good fats are essential and not to be avoided. It's important to understand the difference between good and bad fats (see page 247). Understanding labels is key to making sure you are buying and eating the best possible health-giving foods.

Sugar

Sugar is a drug—it's addictive!

Apart from being a highly toxic and harmful substance, sugar is responsible, at least in part, for the following:
• Weight gain/obesity
• Tooth decay and gum disease
• Diabetes
• Mood swings
• Depression
• Anxiety
• Hormonal imbalances
• Depletion of nutrients from deep within the body
• Premature aging of the body and skin
• Dullness and congestion within the skin
• Low energy levels

Daily consumption of sugar produces a continuously alkaline over-acid condition. Consequently, minerals are required from deep within the body tissues, such as bones and teeth, in order to buffer the acidic environment and rectify the imbalance. So much calcium is taken from the bones and teeth that decay and general weakening begin. Consuming refined sugars eventually affects the whole body.

On top of that, a high sugar diet stops leptin, the hormone that inhibits hunger when you are full, from working properly, so when we consume sugar we have a big tendency to overeat.

Somehow we have to find a way of including treats and a little sweetness in our lives without doing the damage. We can achieve this by finding delicious, natural,

health-giving alternatives. Raw honey, pure maple syrup, raw chocolate, and fruit are great sugar alternatives that provide complex sugars, nourishment, and essential micronutrients to the body without depleting its own resources—and they taste amazing.

Water

Water is essential to a healthy mind, body, and soul. Our bodies are over 60 percent water.

We need water in order to think clearly and flush the build up of toxins from within the body. Our brains are over 70 percent water and require a daily dose of pure clean water from foods, herbal teas, and drinking water in order to function well and think clearly. The signs of dehydration are constipation, headaches, tiredness, and the feeling of hunger. Often when you think you're hungry, your body is actually trying to tell you that it's dehydrated. It's important to drink either filtered water, pure spring, or mineral water to receive the best benefits without any of the chemicals or additives in straight tap water. However, bottled mineral water is often stored in plastic bottles that contain BPA (Bisphenol A), which is an accumulative chemical that has been found to drastically increase the levels of estrogen within the body, regardless of whether you are female or male. In males, this can cause prostate cancer and lowered sperm count. In females, it can cause breast cancer. In children and infants, BPA has been shown to promote hyperactivity. In addition, plastic bottles are insanely bad for the environment. A great way around this is to use BPA-free plastic or metal or glass bottles that you can use again and again by filling up with filtered water or spring water. This is not only cheaper, but its better for the environment and for your body.

Fruit and vegetables

In the past, most produce was left to fully mature before being harvested and used within a short distance of its source. Nowadays most commercially produced grains, fruits, and some vegetables are harvested before they are fully ripened, which inevitably means reduced nourishment. For example, produce picked early doesn't develop as many sunlight-related nutrients such as anthocyanins and polyphenols, compounds that give fruit their color and flavor and which protect against DNA damage, brain cell deterioration, and cancer. The best way around this is to grow and/ or source fruits and vegetables that are as local and seasonal as possible. This kind of produce is most often found in farmers markets, in certain "what's in season" sections in the supermarket, or on your neighbor's apple tree!

Grains, nuts, and seeds—to soak or not to soak

Grains, nuts, beans, and seeds are rich in enzymes. However, unsoaked or unsprouted, they also contain enzyme inhibitors such as phytic acid, a substance present in the bran of all grains, nuts, and seeds. It inhibits the absorbtion of calcium, magnesium, iron, copper, and zinc, and makes them hard to digest. Sprouting or soaking neutralizes the enzyme inhibitors present in all grains, nuts, and seeds, making them easy to digest and much more nutritious—this has always been done in traditional cultures. By soaking and/or sprouting, you are in effect mimicking the process of germination. This increases the enzyme activity by as much as six times, making them much more nutritionally valuable. I always soak my grains, nuts, and seeds. Homemade sprouts are fun to make and so delicious added to salads and sandwiches.

Detox your pantry

It's a great idea to detox your pantry. Clear out anything that doesn't support your health. That way, you won't be tempted by toxic snacks when you're hungry or tired. Having only delicious and health-giving ingredients in your fridge and pantry will help you to stay on your path of eating nourishing, wonderful food.

Caffeine

Caffeine is a stimulant. An excess (more than two cups a day) can place a huge amount of stress on the adrenal glands, causing your body to produce excess amounts of the hormones adrenaline and cortisol. These hormones help the body respond to stress and, when there is too much of it flooding your system, it will make the body store fat. Too much caffeine can also contribute to cellulite, as it impedes the circulation of nutrients to the skin, also depleting the skin of important nutrients like calcium and vitamin B. Since caffeine is a diuretic, it can make you dehydrated and contribute to water retention in your body. It's not all bad though; having one (no more than one) cup of good-quality organic coffee a day can give the body antioxidants and help aid digestion. The same goes for green tea. Because it contains less caffeine than coffee, you can drink more of it, and it is much higher in the antioxidants that are so good for the body. Avoid decaffeinated drinks completely, because they have been highly processed.

Portion tip

So you're being super healthy and feeling great for it, but make sure you're aware of portion sizes—use your hand as guide.
Palm = Proteins: this will include fish, poultry, beans, tofu and tempeh.
Fist = Carbohydrate: whole grains and rice etc.
Hand = Vegetables: a spread hand is a good portion (the greener the better).
Thumb = Fats: good, healthy fats.

LIFESTYLE

If you want to achieve a healthier lifestyle in a realistic way, remember the ratio of 90:10. If you follow your healthy approach 90 percent of the time, you can allow yourself the remaining 10 percent to relax and enjoy yourself. This means you can still enjoy treats, but try to make sure they stay in the 10 percent and don't become habit. You should never just write a day off and think that because you have slipped up, you might as well let your healthy approach go. Life is constantly moving forward, so leave your moment of weakness behind and move forward.

Say no to the ready-made meal

Processed food is the enemy because it has been altered from its natural state. Foods that were once nutritious have been so highly processed that they then have to have an array of different artificial ingredients added back into them to make them taste good. Bulking agents and fillers mean that processed food is cheaper to buy, and added preservatives mean that it will last a long time sitting on the supermarket shelf.

They then no longer contain any of the good micronutrients and enzymes our bodies need. Although these convenience foods can seem tempting, there are so many other ways that are quick, simple, cheap, and delicious to feed yourself and/or your family. Check out the recipes in this book to see how easy it is to make healthy and delicious fast food.

No fad diets

Most people (including all three of us) have tried strict diets and crazy hardcore exercise plans... do they work? Yes, they do initially. But are they sustainable? No! Does the weight you lose always come back? Yes! Are you enjoying the exercise? No. Is it healthy? No.

Trying to follow a strict diet or full-on training regime can be super tough. You go for it one hundred percent with the best intentions. You start to see results and you think that there is no stopping you... but life gets in the way. You have a stressful day, the kids are sick, you're behind with a major deadline at work and you're exhausted, so you skip your gym session. You throw a pizza in the oven and, since you've blown the diet anyway, you down half a bottle of wine, too. In one quick moment your great routine has fallen apart. Then you spend the rest of the night feeling guilty. You feel like all the hard work you have put in over the last few weeks is for nothing, and you slip back into your old routine.

Not only does your body start to yo-yo in weight, but also it puts a huge amount of stress on your body's metabolism. Find your balance. Small changes make a big difference; don't try and do it all at once.

Chewing

Taking your time to chew your food is seriously important. Chewing makes saliva that breaks down your food so it can be digested properly. If you eat too fast and swallow lumps of unchewed food, it will sit in your stomach undigested for a long time, causing bloating and gas. If you eat a nutritious meal and don't chew it properly, a lot of the vitamins and minerals contained in the food won't be released. Take your time during every meal and chew each mouthful at least 20 times. For a flatter, happier tummy, it's time to chew.

Alcohol

Alcohol is a popular way to cope with stress. It's relaxing, it's legal, and it's everywhere. But alcohol is the simplest and most fattening sugar of them all. Full of empty calories, it's super toxic and causes damage to almost every part of the body, from the internal organs to the skin. Drinking alcohol decreases your muscle mass, which will leave your body soft and out of shape. Being aware of the side effects of alcohol is important, so it doesn't become the go-to stress relief at the end of each day.

Moderation is key, so the occasional glass of red wine or a cooling G&T is fine. It's not about denying yourself the ritual or pleasure, it's about replacing it with delicious and health-giving alternatives.

pH levels

The aim is to keep acid low. Your body is constantly working to keep your pH levels in balance and we can help it along by eating the right things. Acid-forming foods like refined sugars, meat, wheat, and processed foods aren't good for the body. An acidic body is like a magnet for disease, sickness, cancer, and aging. Alkaline foods keep your body healthy and functioning properly. High alkaline foods include most vegetables, wheatgrass, almonds, some fruits, and seeds.

Stop counting calories

We've got to step away from the idea that all calories are created equal. They are not. Here's a great example: take one Mars bar and one and a half avocados; they have roughly the same number of calories. However, the way in which your body processes these two foods couldn't be more different. When you consume the Mars bar, your body effectively recognizes it as poison—your built-in alarm systems kick into gear and a chemical process happens that takes the poisons out of your blood stream and into your fat cells. On the other hand, when you eat an avocado, your body recognizes it as a nourishing food source. It is able to absorb all those wonderful calories and turn them into cellular building blocks and life-giving energy for your body to function properly. It then pushes anything it doesn't require through the digestive system and out the other end.

Mars bars = toxins = fat = cravings = moodiness.

Avocado = energy = nourishment = satisfaction = happiness.

It's not about counting calories, but making sure the calories you are eating are the good ones.

FATS
The Good, the Bad & the Ugly

The human brain is about 60 percent fat (dry weight). Every membrane of every cell and every organelle inside of cells are made of fats. Many hormones, neurotransmitters, and other active substances in the body are made of fats. Fats are extremely important in our diet. The big question is: which fats?

Let us first tell you about margarines, butter replacements, "spreadable" vegetable oils, shortenings, and many other artificial fats. They are hydrogenated to increase their shelf life and to make them the right consistency. You can find hydrogenated oils in most processed foods, such as chocolate, ice cream, cookies, cakes, breads, pastries, frozen meals, chips, etc. Hydrogenation is a process of adding hydrogen molecules to the chemical structure of oils under high pressure at a very high temperature

(250–400°F) in the presence of nickel, aluminum, and sometimes other heavy metals. Remnants of these metals stay in the hydrogenated oils. Nickel and aluminum are both heavy metals, adding to the general toxic load that the body has to work hard to get rid of. Heavy metals, particularly aluminum, have been linked to many degenerative conditions, including Alzheimer's disease and dementia. But that is not the main problem with hydrogenated oils. Hydrogenation changes the chemical structure of the oils, producing a whole host of very harmful fats, more commonly known as "trans fats." Trans-fatty acids are very similar in their structure to their natural counterparts, but they are somewhat back to front. Because of their similarity, they occupy the place of essential fats in the body while being unable to do their job, making cells in a way disabled. All organs and tissues in the body are affected. For example, trans fats have great immune-suppressing ability, playing a detrimental role in many different functions of the immune system. They have been implicated in diabetes and neurological conditions, and they interfere with pregnancy, conception, the normal production of hormones... the list is long.

Fats are essential, but which ones should we consume, and how? Fatty acids keep our hair and skin glowing and support our brains and organs. Fats also help us to absorb fat-soluble vitamins that we want from the vegetables we eat. Essential fatty acids are just that—essential!

• Fat enhances the flavor and texture of food.

• Fat provides us with fuel throughout the day.

• Fat boosts brain power.

The important thing to remember

is that we should only consume fats that are in their natural state, without processing them. Oils must be cold-pressed and raw. Eat fats as nature intended them and you will not go wrong.

For searing, browning & pan-frying (cold-pressed and/or raw)
• Safflower oil
• Sunflower oil
• Ghee
• Coconut oil
• Peanut oil
• Goose/duck fat

Sautéing & oven-baking
• Safflower oil
• Sunflower oil
• Ghee
• Coconut oil
• Peanut oil
• Goose fat/duck fat
• Olive oil
• Canola oil
• Grapeseed oil
• Sesame oil

Salad dressings, marinades, dips
• Walnut oil
• Pumpkin seed oil
• Avocado oil
• Flax seed oil
• Extra virgin olive oil
• Sesame seed oil
• Hazelnut oil
• Canola oil

Oils for supplementation
• A good nut/seed oil blend—2:1 ratio of omega-3 to 6 fatty acids
• Cod liver oil
• Fish oil with a higher ratio of fatty acids EPA or DHA

Love, Holly & Amber xx

NOURISH WEEK

The aim for this week is to nourish your body from the inside out. Be gentle and kind to yourself, and take time out of your busy life to focus on you. The Nourish Week can be a warm-up to the Cleanse & Tone Week (pages 250–251), giving you a 2-week program (which we do ourselves)—it feels amazing! The idea of a Nourish Week is not to go on some crazy elimination diet where we end up feeling awful and have loads of withdrawal symptoms, but to simply really nourish your body so you feel energized, calm, replenished, and recharged.
Love, Sadie xx

Monday	Morning: 6–10 Sun Salutations (pages 132–133) Evening: 5–10 minutes of Following the Breath (page 142)
Tuesday	A 20-minute mindful walk/jog, really being present in the moment
Wednesday	Morning: 6–10 Sun Salutations (pages 132–133) Evening: 5–10 minutes of Following the Breath (page 142)
Thursday	A 20-minute mindful walk/jog, really being present in the moment
Friday	Morning: 10 Sun Salutations (pages 132–133) Evening: 5–10 minutes of Following the Breath (page 142)
Saturday	A 20-minute mindful walk/jog, really being present in the moment
Sunday	Morning: 5–10 minutes of Following the Breath (page 142)

This eating plan can be adapted to meet certain dietary requirements. If you're vegetarian, swap the fish or chicken for a different veggie option in the main dish section. If you don't eat grains or dairy, simply replace the milk or kefir in the smoothies with full-fat coconut milk or almond milk and use coconut cream or yogurt for the granola or fruit salad. I am sure there will be meals that you won't want to try, or maybe you'll just need a break. If that's the case, just try to make wise decisions and avoid sugar and refined carbs. Remember, the more you nourish yourself, the less you will need the bad stuff.

Love, Amber xx

	Breakfast	*Snack*	*Lunch*	*Snack*	*Dinner*
Monday	Banana & Almond Smoothie (page 17)	An herbal tea and any snack from the list below	Nourish Bowl (page 66)	An herbal tea and any snack from the list below	Puy Lentils with Wilted Spinach (page 53) and a piece of pan-fried fish*
Tuesday	Poached Eggs with Cauliflower Toasts (page 34)	An herbal tea and any snack from the list below	Nourish Bowl (page 66)	An herbal tea and any snack from the list below	Japanese Chicken (page 68) with Smashed Cucumber Salad (page 56) and quinoa or brown rice*
Wednesday	Som Tum Pollamai (page 47) with your favorite yogurt	An herbal tea and any snack from the list below	Nourish Bowl (page 66)	An herbal tea and any snack from the list below	Spring "Spaghetti" with Kale Pesto & Arugula Flowers (page 80)*
Thursday	Blackberry, Rose & Raw Chocolate Smoothie (page 14)	An herbal tea and any snack from the list below	Nourish Bowl (page 66)	An herbal tea and any snack from the list below	My Mom's Veg Chili (page 79)*
Friday	A smoothie of your choice (pages 14–17)	An herbal tea and any snack from the list below	Nourish Bowl (page 66)	An herbal tea and any snack from the list below	Lemon & Sumac Chicken (page 70) and Quinoa with a Rainbow of Jewels (page 62)*
Saturday	Poached Eggs with Cauliflower Toasts (page 34)	An herbal tea and any snack from the list below	A soup of your choice (pages 50–52)	An herbal tea and any snack from the list below	Japanese Brown Rice Bowl and Kimchi (page 67) or Baked Haddock with Ginger (page 76)*
Sunday	Coconut & Banana Pancakes (page 33)	An herbal tea and any snack from the list below	Late lunch/early dinner: Mexican Feast (pages 72–73)		

* You can follow any dinner with an optional dessert from the Sweet Tooth section (pages 82–103)

Snacks

Choose from the following:
- A handful of soaked raw almonds
- 1 orange
- 2 medjool dates
- 1 or 2 Spiced Chocolate & Sweet Potato Brownies (page 96), depending on size
- A few Coconut & Apricot Bliss Balls (page 91)
- A handful of blueberries

CLEANSE & TONE WEEK

The aim for this week is to cleanse the body from the inside and to really push and challenge your body from the outside. The Cleanse & Tone week is great to do if you really want to feel great for an event, a vacation, or special occasion coming up. Pick a workout program week that suits your level of fitness.
Love, Holly xx

Monday	• Warm Up (pages 206–207) • Workout 1 from program of your choice (pages 211–241) • Stretches
Tuesday	• Warm Up (pages 206–207) • 15 minutes jumping rope • One Tabata Workout (page 242) • Stretches
Wednesday	• Warm Up (pages 206–207) • Workout 2 from program of your choice (pages 211–241) • Stretches
Thursday	• 30-minute jog • Stretches
Friday	• Warm Up (pages 206–207) • Workout 3 from program of your choice (pages 211–241) • Stretches
Saturday	• 30-minute jog • Stretches
Sunday	• Warm Up (pages 206–207) • 15 minutes jumping rope • One Tabata Workout (page 242) • Stretches

This eating plan is a little bit stricter than The Nourish Week. The best way to make it through each of these plans is to do a little planning and get yourself organized with at least a day's worth of food ready to go in the fridge and pantry. Try to go through this part of gathering, shopping, and preparing in a positive way. Don't think of it as chore, but as part of the creative, learning, and growing process we all have to go through to love and nourish ourselves.

Love, Amber xx

	Breakfast	*Snack*	*Lunch*	*Dinner*
Monday to Friday	A Green Juice (page 21) or a smoothie (pages 14–17) and/or Som Tum Pollamai (page 47) with yogurt or A bowl of fresh fruit and a sprinkle of Grain-free Granola (page 40)	An herbal tea and any snack from the list below	A soup of your choice (pages 50–52) or a Nourish Bowl (page 66)	Choose from the dinners listed in Nourish Week (page 249), but try to avoid carbs and late-night eating
Saturday	Poached Eggs with Cauliflower Toasts (page 34)	An herbal tea and any snack from the list below	A soup of your choice (pages 50–52) or a Nourish Bowl (page 66)	Japanese Chicken (page 68) with Smashed Cucumber Salad (page 56) and a green leafy salad
Sunday	A Green Juice (page 21) or a smoothie (pages 14–17) and/or Som Tum Pollamai (page 47) with yogurt or A bowl of fresh fruit and a sprinkle of Grain-free Granola (page 40)	An herbal tea and any snack from the list below	Late lunch/early dinner: Mexican Feast (pages 72–73) or Lemon & Sumac Chicken (page 70) and Quinoa with a Rainbow of Jewels (page 62)	

Snacks

Choose from the following:

- A handful of soaked raw almonds
- 1 orange
- A handful of Kale Crisps (page 108)
- A few Coconut & Apricot Bliss Balls (page 91)
- A handful of blueberries
- Some raw vegetables with Hummus (page 107)

INDEX

ACKNOWLEDGMENTS

Amber

There are a lot of people that I would like to show my thanks and love and gratitude to…

Firstly, I would like to thank my son: you are a constant source of love and inspiration and you keep me going. Thank you for all your patience and support; you really are the love of my life.

I would like to thank all the beautiful, talented, strong, incredible women in my life who have given me endless support and love and strength along the way to stay true to myself and keep going when things have not been easy: Vanessa Cooke, India Waters, Nandi Boyle, Beshlie Mckelvie, Nicola Guinness, Ali Allen—you have all made me who I am today and I love you all.

Thank you to Rosie Scott for her amazing support and guidance and for her endless encouragement in all areas of my life. You are amazing and I love you.

To Lucinda Carey: you are an amazing woman with so much to give. You have been such a huge support and I have so much love and respect for you and your beautiful children whom I love and adore. Thank you for your love along the way.

To Ieva Imsa and Ivor Guest, thank you for your support and strength.

You have been pillars in a sometimes rocky landscape. You are an inspiration and a joy to know.

Thank you to all the women in my family who have shared their love of food with me, midnight feasts and leisurely breakfasts, Sunday roasts, and salads freshly picked from the garden. Vivien, Marion, and Rachel, you rock—you're the best aunties anyone could ask for. Thank you Maida, I will never forget your crackling and your ginger nut cookies and cups of steaming hot Milo on a cold winter's day.

Thank you mom for growing the best garden full of the most amazing food that has spawned a life long obsession with food. I will always steal the first peaches, and rummage through the berry patch for the first berries—hope you don't mind!

I would also like to thank Sadie Frost and Holly Davidson for sharing this journey with me, for having the patience and love to keep going and plow through. You are both amazing and you are both an inspiration to me. Many more adventures to come.

Sadie

I would like to thank all my brothers and sisters and my Ma and Pa! My four beautiful children for keeping me young at heart.

Also thanks to all my gurus with whom I've studied yoga: Nadia Narain, Stewart Gilchrist, Bryony Bird, Luiz Veiga, and the beautiful Hortense Suleyman. Hugh Poulton for showing me balance. Dan Burt for keeping me stretched and toned in Pilates.

Thanks to Yehudi Gordon for being there spiritually and with all the mind, body, and soul I could have ever have needed. Nish Joshi for the acupuncture, healing, and Zest and of course the lovely Chip and Heidi Somers who helped me through some of my most difficult times.

Also for showing me how it's done: Kate Moss, Jemima French, Emma Comley, Rose Ferguson, Fran Cutler, Collette Cooper, and Grimmy and all my other spiritual fairies.

I would also like to thank all the fantastic teachers at Transcendental Meditation in London and Andy Puddicome from Head Space.

A big acknowledgment to the beautiful and spirited Zoe Grace and Jade Davidson for having the most lovely soul ever!

Holly

I would like to thank each and every one of my clients. You are all the reason why this book took flight. Thank you for your help, support, ideas, and encouragement; you are all a daily inspiration to me. A special thanks to Sardia Khan and Sienna Guillory.

Julie Lane, you are my guardian angel and words can't thank you enough for your help and time, and for taking me under your wing.

To Angelo Di Muro, thank you for setting me on the right track, for keeping your cool, and for your fantastic organization and planning.

I would like to thank all the mentors in my life. Their incredible knowledge and passion to teach has given me the hunger to learn more.

A special thanks to my first yoga teacher Gerry Ross, your smile and energy for life is contagious, and to Stewart Gilchrist, a magnificent guru who continues to challenge my body and mind.

Thank you, Dai Master Rafael Nieto, for making me strong and disciplined. And to all the senseis at Xen-Do who have taught me over the years. And Steve Harrison a great teacher, thank you for passing on your passion.

To my sister, Jade Davidson. I thank you with all my heart for your endless kindness, patience, wisdom, and friendship. You are my shining star.

Thank you to all of my gorgeous family. Especially my niece and nephews Billy, Fin, Raff, Sean, Iris, and Rudy for always making me smile.

Thank you to all the amazing friends I have around me. I love you all very dearly: Helen Bouillet, Jade Bevan, Natalie Ferstendik, Shelley Conn, Vicki Ballington, Bebhinn Gleeson, Triana Terry. And an extra big hug and love to Ania Sowinski.

I'd like to send special thanks to my second family, The Baldwins—Tom, Rebecca, Frankie, and Arthur—for your continuous support, love and friendship.

My NY boy, I want to thank you for your patience and support.

And of course a huge thanks to Sadie and Amber. You both have been pillars of strength and inspiration in my life. And to be able to have shared writing this book with you both has been such a wonderful journey. Thank you!

From the 3 of us

Firstly we would all like to thank Kyle, for her belief in this project, for her unwavering support, and for cracking the whip when necessary— we would be nothing without you. Thank you for pulling this book together and giving us the support and guidance to shine. You have been utterly amazing, thank you!!!!

We would like to thank Heather Holden-Brown, our collective agent, for supporting us through this project and guiding us when we needed it. You have been a dream agent and we couldn't have got this far without you.

Thank you to David Loftus for bringing our vision to life, for your beautiful pictures and amazing eye. Thank you for all your hard work and support. You have given beauty and elegance to our project.

Thank you to Shiv, Fabiola, Jackie, and Lilly for making us all gorgeous and beautiful and confident. You are all amazing, talented ladies.

A special thank you goes out to Rukmini Iyer for your support and help in the kitchen.

Additional thanks to the following PR Agencies and suppliers for generously supplying the equipment and outfits used in this book:
Asquith London, Beshlie McKelvie (www.beshlie.com), Chinti and Parker, Didi Ilse Jewellery, Fabi-Atelier, Goodley PR, Karla Otto London, Isabel Marant, The Meditator, MIH Jeans, Nike, Zadig et Voltaire.